GIRLFRIEND MATERIAL

For the little girl who was once terrified and afraid of who she was, and to all of the fierce women, past and present, who lifted her up, cheered her on and showed her what a gentle but powerful rebellion can look like.

When you persevere, trust the journey, and allow yourself to truly feel, *anything* is possible.

Rosie Turner

GIRLFRIEND MATERIAL

An honest guide
to dating women and
owning your identity

GREEN TREE
LONDON · OXFORD · NEW YORK · NEW DELHI · SYDNEY

GREEN TREE
Bloomsbury Publishing Plc
50 Bedford Square, London, WC1B 3DP, UK
Bloomsbury Publishing Ireland Limited,
29 Earlsfort Terrace, Dublin 2, D02 AY28, Ireland

BLOOMSBURY, GREEN TREE and the Green Tree logo are trademarks of Bloomsbury Publishing Plc

First published in Great Britain 2026
Copyright © Rosie Turner 2026

Rosie Turner has asserted her right under the Copyright, Designs and Patents Act, 1988, to be identified as Author of this work.

Every reasonable effort has been made to trace copyright holders of material reproduced in this book, but if any have been inadvertently overlooked the publishers would be glad to hear from them. For legal purposes the Acknowledgements on p. 249 constitute an extension of this copyright page.

All rights reserved. No part of this publication may be: i) reproduced or transmitted in any form, electronic or mechanical, including photocopying, recording or by means of any information storage or retrieval system without prior permission in writing from the publishers; or ii) used or reproduced in any way for the training, development or operation of artificial intelligence (AI) technologies, including generative AI technologies. The rights holders expressly reserve this publication from the text and data mining exception as per Article 4(3) of the Digital Single Market Directive (EU) 2019/790

Bloomsbury Publishing Plc does not have any control over, or responsibility for, any third-party websites referred to or in this book. All internet addresses given in this book were correct at the time of going to press. The author and publisher regret any inconvenience caused if addresses have changed or sites have ceased to exist but can accept no responsibility for any such changes.

A catalogue record for this book is available from the British Library.

Library of Congress Cataloguing-in-Publication data has been applied for.

ISBN: HB: 978-1-3994-2610-7; eBook: 978-1-3994-2609-1; ePDF: 978-1-3994-2608-4

2 4 6 8 10 9 7 5 3 1

Text design by D.R. Ink
Typeset by Lumina Datamatics Ltd

Printed and bound in Great Britain by Clays Ltd, Elcograf S.p.A

To find out more about our authors and books visit www.bloomsbury.com and sign up for our newsletters.
For product safety related questions contact productsafety@bloomsbury.com

Please note that names marked * in the book have been changed to protect individuals' privacy.

Contents

Introduction	**6**
1. Coming out	**11**
2. Labels	**48**
3. Connections	**67**
4. Dating	**87**
5. Sex	**133**
6. Relationships	**164**
7. The grey area of love	**205**
8. Closing thoughts	**238**
Acknowledgements	**244**
Sources	**246**

Introduction

Let's get real for a hot minute. When you first start questioning your sexuality or begin the process of coming out, no one hands you a guidebook. There's no welcome pack, no survival manual, no road map explaining what the hell to do next, and honestly, the fact that one doesn't exist feels like a crime.

But if there's one thing I've learned, it's this: waiting around for someone else to give you permission won't get you very far.

So, I decided to write one.

Welcome to my no-bullshit, funny, emotional, awkward, affirming and deeply needed guide, which I wish I'd had when I was figuring it all out. If you've been searching for something that cuts through the confusion, makes you feel seen and helps you laugh through the chaos, then this book is for you.

It's part coming-out survival manual, part guidebook (yes: sex ed, technique *and* emotional literacy), part psychology deep-dive and part collection of real-life stories – the chaotic, the messy and the moving.

Vague advice, tired clichés or those recycled '10 signs she's into you' lists from days gone by just don't cut it any more. We're craving something real. Something that answers the questions that actually keep us up at night, like:

- *How do I know if she actually likes me?*
- *What if I'm already in a relationship while figuring this all out?*
- *How do I make queer friends who truly get me?*
- *How can I be incredible in bed?*
- *And seriously – how the hell do women even flirt with each other?!*

Inside, we're unpacking it all: the grey area between friendship and something more, how to hit on someone without looking like a d*ck, what

INTRODUCTION

healthy intimacy actually looks like and why queer friendships are the emotional backbone of so many of our lives. And it's not just me. You'll also hear from other queer women, as well as from experts in love, sex, psychology and identity whose research I've included along the way.

This book is rooted in everything I've learned as a queer woman, a content creator and a community builder who has spent years carving out spaces (both online and in real life) where LGBTQIA+ (lesbian, gay, bisexual, transgender, queer, intersex, asexual or other), women can feel safe, seen and celebrated. From the thousands of DMs I've received, to the hilarious and heartbreaking stories I've shared, to the viral tutorials (yes, *that* video on how to go down on a woman that racked up over 13 million views on TikTok and earned me more than a few curious stares in public – you're welcome), I've seen first-hand how deeply we're craving honest, unfiltered conversations about love, sex, identity and connection. And let's be real: we need to be able to laugh about it too. Because it's nothing if not gloriously, beautifully chaotic.

So, who am I?

I'm Rosie, and you might know me from the internet (@rosieturnerdaily), where I've spent years creating content around self-acceptance, embracing the joy in life and sticking two unapologetic fingers up at the societal norms that try to box us in. Helping people find their confidence, connect with their identity and laugh along the way isn't just my brand – it's who I am.

My mission is simple: to help you feel more connected, more confident and more in love with your life, exactly as you are.

I'm not a qualified therapist (though, judging by my bookshelf, you might think otherwise), so I can't give clinical advice, but what I *can* offer is lived experience, stories of near breakdowns, hilarious missteps, hard-earned lessons and the beautiful mess that is becoming yourself.

I'll bring you truth, humour and a grounded perspective from someone who's walked through the hard stuff and come out the other side with a pretty decent emotional toolkit in one hand (and a glass of wine in the other).

The reason why I've written this book, and in turn care so much about what lies inside it, is because I know exactly what it feels like to be completely *without* guidance. To be unsure of yourself, to feel different in a way that's hard to put into words and to carry the fear that so many of us feel: that there's something wrong with us.

When I was 15, a year before I was meant to sit my final exams, I made the difficult decision to leave high school early. It wasn't just one thing that led me there, but a mix of many: bullying; the responsibility of caring for my mum, who was unwell at the time; the grief of losing people I loved; and a tangle of mental health struggles that slowly wrapped themselves around me, pulling me into an incredibly dark and isolating place.

It was one of the hardest periods of my life, and right in the middle of it, when everything felt uncertain, I was also beginning to question my identity and sexuality.

I had no blueprint, no community, no road map. Just questions, fear and yet a stubborn, quiet voice inside me that whispered, *There has to be more.*

And there was – I just hadn't found it yet.

In those 12 months away from the noise of the world outside, I learned a lot in the silence. About who I was. About who I wanted to become. But most of all, I learned this: you can't control the cards you're dealt in life, but you can control your story.

You can choose how you frame your experiences, and how you use them – not to define you, but to propel you forwards, rather than keep you stuck in the past. And I want to share that with you too.

My mum has always reminded me that being different isn't something to hide – it's something to celebrate. She named me after a wild rose she saw growing in a hedgerow days after I was born: beautifully soft yet impossible to tame. She had no idea then how perfectly that would describe the woman I'd become. Back then, I didn't feel strong. But looking back now I can see that I was quietly building a foundation, without even realising it, that would one day allow me to live authentically, build a community and help others do the same.

I might not have seen a future for myself at the time, but over the years – through educating myself, doing the hard introspective work and connecting with others – I have found my voice. I've shared my story online for others to read, created content that makes people feel less alone and started building the kind of community I'd once desperately needed and longed for.

It's a community that extends to all corners of my life and one that I hope you will now learn from, and feel a part of, through reading this book.

So wherever you are on your journey, whether you're scared, curious, questioning or healing, I hope these pages remind you that you are *not* broken, weird or behind.

You're just beginning.

I'm not here to tell you how to live your life. That would be boring. I'm here to offer a gentle (and hopefully funny) guide to help you through the messy middle. And it's not just me talking – this book is shaped by the voices of queer women from all walks of life: friends, family, people I love – content creators, community builders and soul-healers. The ones I've cried, laughed and shared many 2a.m. kitchen-table therapy sessions with.

To honour them, I've included a 'queer voices' feature throughout the book that spotlights their thoughts and experiences.

There's no one way to be queer. No perfect path to follow. But there *is* power in knowing you're not alone.

A note on the text

Throughout the book, I use the term 'woman' to describe people who self-identify as such. This includes trans women, nonbinary people, those who identify as gender expansive and anyone whose identity aligns with womanhood in a way that resonates for them.

Your gender identity and sexuality are yours to define, and however you exist in the world, you are valid, welcome and seen here.

For the sake of clarity and ease in writing, much of this book refers to interactions between two women using she/her pronouns. But please know that love, desire, confusion, joy, heartbreak and healing are not bound by gender, and the core themes in these pages – connection, identity and self-acceptance – are for anyone who sees themselves reflected in this journey.

To protect individuals' privacy, names marked * have been changed.

Please also note that language can change and labels can be complicated. I've devoted a whole chapter to labels and provide some simple definitions of common terms on p. 54, based on current trends and information, but this may change in the future.

The experiences I've included are as expansive as I could make them, drawn from the stories of people in my life and community, and shaped with care, love and intention.

While no book can hold every experience, I've tried my hardest to make this one feel like a home for as many of us as possible.

Because at its core, *Girlfriend Material* is about giving you permission.

Permission to question, permission to want, permission to take up space, to mess up, to try again and to laugh at yourself along the way.

Whether you're figuring things out at the age of 16, 36 or 56, you deserve to live your life out loud.

(And yes, it's also, somewhat cheekily, about how to become great *girlfriend material* ... which, let's be honest, we all want to know!)

Whoever you are, however you identify and wherever you are on your path, I'm so glad you're here.

So let's unlearn the rules we were never meant to follow and build something new together – honest, unfiltered and *full* of heart.

I'm genuinely excited to see what thoughts, questions or feelings come up for you as you explore the chapters ahead.

I'm slightly less excited about having to reach out to my entire dating history to let them know they're now part of this unpacking journey.

[coughs awkwardly]
Shall we begin?

ONE

Coming out

The phrase 'coming out' gives me the ick.

Why are we still having to broadcast who we want to hook up with, like a cringe manager giving a drunken speech at an office party?

[taps glass]

'Hello everyone, I'd just like to say that I won't be shagging Paul from Accounts any more; I actually prefer Katrina on the front desk . . . just thought you'd all like to know.'

When you really think about it, that's essentially what coming out still feels like: making an unnecessary announcement about something that should be private. It's no one else's business how we live our lives, yet society still acts like it has the right to weigh in, no matter how far we've come.

For many of us, coming out is the first step to fully acknowledging our sexual identity and starting a new chapter in our lives, but we often forget that the process of coming out has two parts. It's not just about sharing how you feel with *others* but acknowledging, accepting and embracing your identity with *yourself* first.

And self-acceptance can be the hardest stage to go through in your identity journey (which is why it's touched on here and explored in more depth in chapter 3). The reason for the struggle is that we're often alone in our thoughts, trying hard to navigate a time that can be filled with mood changes, uncertainty, internalised homophobia, shame, envy, excitement, anxiety and for many, denial, to name a few.

That's why, in this first chapter, we're diving into both sides of coming out: to yourself, and to others. Think of this as your 'coming out 101' roadmap. We'll look at:

- How to come out to yourself – to help guide you through the experience and answer some of the most common questions you've been burning to ask.
- The invisible barriers that might stop you from coming out to yourself and others, such as denial and emotional paralysis and even internalised homophobia.
- Finally, I'll gift you with a five-step road map for how to come out to yourself and, if you want to, others.

This chapter is for *everyone*, and I really want to emphasise that, no matter your age or relationship status. Whether you're single, married, figuring it out, in the middle of a transition or just feeling totally f*cking lost, I've got you.

Coming out to yourself

I want to start this section with a little tough love. Think of it as a gentle, but honest, wake-up call. Not to rush you into accepting your feelings before you're ready, but because these truths often go unspoken, and someone needs to say them, so here I am.

The journey to truly understanding yourself ultimately sits with *you*.

You can bring in as many therapists, counsellors, coaches, friends, family or colleagues as you like to help unpack your emotions and feelings (which I highly recommend) but at the end of the day, the decision about how you live your life and show up each day is yours alone.

Once you recognise this, it's a game changer.

Coming out to yourself is often the hardest part of the acceptance journey. It's scary to step into something new that you don't fully understand yet. It also means confronting and working through behaviours and limiting beliefs that may have held you back for years.

In the period leading up to my coming out, I joked with friends about how low I felt, but I couldn't quite name the reason for that joylessness.

It was like wandering through a house with all the lights switched off, hoping something would flicker on.

It wasn't until I made the decision to dig deeper and acknowledge that my repressed sexuality was a huge part of how down I felt that things began to change.

Piece by piece, like painting by numbers, I started to see the picture emerge, revealing what might really be going on beneath the surface.

Exploring your sexual or gender identity is never a compartmentalised experience, separate from the rest of your life. It requires looking at yourself fully, asking hard questions, revisiting past experiences, re-evaluating choices and sitting with that uncertainty.

It takes time listening to podcasts, reading books, talking to therapists, friends and even sometimes people you have feelings for (eek). But most importantly, it takes listening to yourself when answers arise, interpreting them honestly and with care, and . . . then choosing to accept what your intuition reveals.

That, to me, is what coming out to yourself really looks like. Yes, it can be confusing, overwhelming and emotionally exhausting, but it's also deeply liberating, and absolutely worth it.

It's never too late

The number one question I get asked when I post advice around coming out online is, 'Have I left it too late?' And the answer simply is: no.

It doesn't matter whether you're 14 or 40, your sexuality and identity aren't dependent on a time or date (although you could piggyback off a birthday or family celebration and save money on the cake and streamers). The timing of when you choose to better understand yourself is entirely your own and if anyone judges you for that, it says more about their own discomfort with growth than yours. Also, more often than not, they're probably quietly wishing they had the courage to do the same.

There *really* is no right or wrong way to come out to yourself or others, but from my own experience and listening to the stories of those around me in the community, I have some top tips I can share to navigate this period well.

Let's dive straight in.

The 'realisation' moment

Let's start at the very beginning, aka the 'realisation' moment. I've had people talk to me about the shame they feel around taking years to come to the realisation that they like women, and how much judgement they've placed on themselves for not doing something about it sooner.

My answer to this is always the same: sometimes you are simply not prepared or at a point in your life to handle hard information or truths. There's a reason why things happen when they do and you have to trust that the timing is right for *you*.

There are loads of things in life we could kick ourselves for not doing sooner. I'd love to have started my own business earlier or studied a different degree at university, but would I change those things? No, because they led me to where I am right now, and where I am now (even though it's been hard at times) is the right place for *me*.

When we start calling parts of our lives mistakes or missed opportunities, we rob ourselves of the chance to appreciate where we are now, and how far we've come, even if it's not perfect.

The journey of understanding and unpacking your sexuality, gender identity or expression is deeply personal, and it looks different for everyone. Some people know from a very young age; others spend years quietly wrestling with a nagging feeling they can't quite name; some take time to explore privately before opening up to anyone else; and then there are people like me, who sense something early on, but push it aside again and again ... until one day, it slaps you in the face, and hiding is no longer an option.

Let's take a look at a few of these different scenarios now:

The ones who already know

Some people have a clear sense of their sexual identity from a very young age. When I first encountered people with this kind of coming-out story, I naively assumed it came with nothing but advantages – and in many ways, it does. Discovering your sexuality early can offer more time and space to explore those feelings, and when you're surrounded by a supportive family or social circle, it can lay a strong foundation for navigating future relationships and conversations with confidence.

But that's not the whole story.

Some people don't have a solid support system growing up. This can make them feel isolated, whether they share their self-knowledge about their sexual identity or not. Knowing who you are from a young age doesn't always mean feeling safe to express it. If they do open up when they're young, and are met with criticism or rejection, this can hit especially hard and leave very deep marks. For some, early experiences of judgement or exclusion can shape how much vulnerability and trust they're willing to risk as adults.

Knowing yourself is powerful. But that knowledge needs to be held in a space of care, safety and compassion, especially when you're still forming your sense of self and learning how to navigate the world.

The ones who have a nagging voice inside

For some people, there's an inner voice that sporadically surfaces at various moments throughout life, gently nudging you to pay attention to something that you may be actively avoiding.

Many people who experience these 'nagging voices' pass them off as anything from general unhappiness and stress to a 'one-off feeling'. But the thing about denying these emotions is that they always tend to grow – to a point where they are often too loud to ignore.

There are many reasons why that inner nagging voice may be uncomfortable to listen to. For example, you might find yourself doubting whether your feelings are valid, not fully understanding the LGBTQ+ space or fearing what might happen if you're honest.

And you're not alone if you're only starting to pay attention to those thoughts later in life. A recent report from Gallup (a global analytics and polling organisation) states that around '10% of LGBTQ+ adults in the US come out after age 30'. In the UK, a generational study of LGBTQI women found that '52% came out after the age of 18', with many older adults not fully coming out until well into their 20s or beyond.

These numbers matter because they remind us that delayed self-recognition isn't a failure, it's common, and deeply human. But when those feelings go unaddressed, they don't disappear. For some, they simmer beneath the surface, eventually spilling out as anger or outward frustration. For others, they become an inward struggle that results in withdrawal, anxiety or depression. On the flip side, others might embrace their new-found sense of self with ease.

It looks different for everyone but thankfully, this book exists and we're unpacking it all together.

The ones where it just slaps you in the face one random Tuesday

Some people might feel perfectly content with their lives, and are walking around in complete bliss, until one afternoon, out of the blue, they suddenly find themselves having romantic feelings for another woman and it shakes up their whole world.

But rather than being a dramatic rebirth, it could probably more accurately be likened to waking up from a hibernation. The thoughts and feelings were likely always there, buried beneath the surface, just waiting for the right moment to rise. Often it only takes just *one* catalyst – something or someone significant or unexpected – to stir them up.

That catalyst can come in many forms: a brief but powerful encounter with someone who turns your world upside down, or a quiet, introspective moment when everything suddenly makes sense.

What matters isn't how it happens, but that it does.

You begin to think in new ways, and the feelings you once pushed aside start to surface with clarity.

This is what the start of coming out to *yourself* looks like.

It's also important to recognise that these realisations don't always end in one 'coming out' moment. Coming into your identity is not always a single event: it can unfold in layers, with new ways of understanding your sexuality continuing to emerge over time.

Here are some stories from other queer women about their coming-out experiences. As you'll see, they vary massively:

COMING OUT

QUEER VOICES

'I came out at 26 years old as bisexual midway through my almost ten-year monogamous marriage to a man. Thankfully, my ex-husband affirmed my queer identity without objectifying or fetishising my attraction to other women. I didn't fully acknowledge or embrace the fact that I liked girls until another friend (who was also in a straight-passing marriage) came out as bi to me.'

'Coming out was definitely a slow burn for me. I came out to my friends first, just casually sleeping with women but still dating men. It wasn't until I fell in love with a woman for the first time that I finally came out to my family. My mom laughed and said, "I know – you have always loved everyone." The rest of the family wasn't so kind and accepting.'

'Falling in love with and marrying a man meant I lived a very straight-presenting life for a long time. It was only when I fell head over heels in lust and infatuation with a woman that I really realised how much those feelings were still there. Coming out in my late 30s felt euphoric. I finally felt that I stepped out from behind a mask and experienced a confidence and self-assuredness that had been missing.'

> **Coming out in my late 30s felt euphoric. I finally felt that I stepped out from behind a mask**

'I realised I liked women during rehearsals for a school French-themed entertainment evening. A girl from the year below came onstage to sing "Chanson d'Amour" in a French maid outfit and I thought, "Oh shit, I like her."'

'I actually realised I liked women when I downloaded an easy-read romance that I thought was about a straight couple but ended up being about a lesbian couple. As I read it and got to the "spicy" parts it just seemed so much more intriguing to me than the [male-female] ones I'd read before, and I really wanted to do those things!'

'For me this is very different, I suspect, from many of the other women in this book. I am a trans lesbian, which means I was assigned male *at birth. I therefore had to deal with the fact that I was in fact attracted to women in a way that perhaps society expected me to be as a child, but also that I was not supposed to be the boy that everyone thought I was. But it was not until I was 36 that I realised that who I am is never changing, and either I do something about it, or I live the rest of my life as a lie.'*

'It was a slow process for me. I'd always been attracted to women since I was very young, but I didn't know anyone in my family or my life who was a lesbian, so I never understood how I could be gay. I didn't look like any of the gay celebrities and it just seemed so normal to feel attracted to beautiful women, but actually just date men.'

MY STORY

The first time *I* truly recognised that I had feelings for another woman was at a Halloween party at university. I was dressed as Barbie and in the space of one evening, realised that maybe it wasn't Ken I wanted to hook up with after all.

Midway through getting ready and putting enough blusher on my cheeks to look like I had alcohol-related rosacea, Becky* wandered into my bedroom, searching for a hairbrush.

She was a friend of a friend, petite with long blonde hair and sparkly eyes. As she stood in my doorway sporting a little beige cardigan and sweatpants, we locked eyes and laughed as she poked fun at me.

'You look nice,' she smirked.

The chemistry was charged.

I handed her the hairbrush. She smiled back at me, disappeared and that was that.

I was now not straight.

COMING OUT

There isn't a way that I can describe the feeling of immediately realising I was into women that night. Even though I'd had suspicions since my mid-teens and dismissed them. Now, I felt a strange mix of being turned on, excited, horrified and feeling like I wanted to die all at once, yet also being extremely at peace with my impending passing.

If someone had held up a microphone to my mind, I imagine my thoughts would have been along the lines of:

F*CK. Why do I think Becky is cute? Becky is a girl. Becky looks a bit like me; do I fancy myself? So I'm a narcissist? Becky is just hot in a friendly way. What does 'hot in a friendly way' mean, Rosie? Were you looking at her weird? Oh my god she thinks you're a creep. You are a creep. Look at your bright pink face and Barbie outfit – this is the literal outfit of a creep. I don't want to have sex with Becky, yuck. If she wanted to kiss me though, I'd be down. OH MY GOD. Did I just say that I want to kiss her? That's gay. I'm gay. I'm going to have to come out to everyone immediately. Didn't I think I was a bit gay before and dismiss it? This makes sense now. I can't marry a woman; is that legal? I don't want to marry Becky. I like having sex with guys. Can I have sex with both? That would be hot if Becky wanted to join. So I'm a lesbian but not? I'm bisexual? I'm straight and just temporarily confused? Oh my god this is a disaster. I look like a clown right now. I am a clown right now. I'm a GAY F*CKING CLOWN. I need a drink.

As comical as the above might sound, the next morning I woke up horrified. All over Facebook were photos of Becky and I dancing, my arms around her, her face close to mine. I rushed to de-tag every piece of incriminating evidence and then lay frozen, staring at the bedroom wall. I knew I couldn't take back what I felt and that I had to finally face it.

The shame that followed in the weeks and months after that night was heavy. Every time I tried to fix it, it felt like I was making things worse, like I was sinking in quicksand. My sense of self had been completely shaken, and it became a dark and isolating place to be. Fear crept in, then took over. It seeped into every part of my life, nagging me with questions I didn't want to answer, but knew I needed to.

The emotional impact of coming out to yourself

The kind of emotional (and somewhat chaotic) spiral I describe in my story is more common than is generally spoken about, especially for women who are just beginning to realise they have feelings for another woman. So I want to highlight some of the thoughts and questions that might surface during this period. You might relate to a few, or maybe all of them, but please remember, just because these thoughts arise, it doesn't mean they'll stay. And if nothing else, I hope you find comfort in knowing you're not alone.

'Am I a creep?'

When we begin to question our sexuality, it can feel like a spotlight is suddenly shining on every interaction we've ever had, especially with other women in our lives. For me, this manifested in re-running past conversations and physical moments in my mind, obsessively checking whether I'd ever behaved in a way that could be seen as predatory or inappropriate. I had internalised the belief that same-sex attraction was somehow wrong or threatening, and I didn't want to make anyone uncomfortable.

Every small thing felt loaded. Brushing my feet against my housemate on the sofa. Accidentally walking in while someone was getting changed. Sharing a bed with a friend, now aware of something they didn't yet know. I was terrified that I might cross a line, or that I already had. I desperately didn't want to be attracted to any of my friends or look at them in a way that was inappropriate, so I became militant with keeping my distance.

But here's the thing: none of this actually helped. What I was doing was quietly shaming myself. I was internalising a false belief that my sexuality somehow made me dangerous, that just *being* queer put the people around me at risk. And that belief is not only untrue, it's harmful.

If you find yourself caught in this spiral, I want you to pause and breathe. You are not a threat. You are not wrong for discovering this part of yourself. Your sexuality doesn't turn you into someone else overnight. It simply *reveals* something true, something human, about who you are and what you want.

Here are a few gentle reminders if this is where you're at:

- **It's OK to feel awkward or uncertain right now.** That doesn't mean you've done anything wrong; it just means you're adjusting to a new truth.
- **You're allowed to set boundaries and take space,** but don't isolate yourself out of shame. Lean on the people you trust.
- **Reframing is powerful.** Instead of asking, 'Did I make them uncomfortable?' ask, 'Was I being respectful, kind and true to myself?'
- **You are not alone.** So many queer women experience this exact internal tug-of-war when they first come out, and it gets easier with time.

The discomfort won't last forever. The shame will ease. And in time, you'll come to see your queerness not as something that sets you apart in a dangerous way, but as something that deepens your capacity for love, empathy and connection. I promise.

'I don't *feel* gay, so how can I *be* gay?'

What does it mean to *feel* an identity? We often don't walk around *feeling* like a woman, a mother or a co-worker. We are simply ourselves.

The same goes for your sexuality. Feeling connected to your identity is a deeply personal journey, and there's no single path or checklist to follow. There is no one way to be 'gay', so however you choose to explore or express that identity is entirely up to you. You might feel called to start fresh and reimagine your life. You might want to carry parts of your past with you – your style, your friendships, your routines – or you might feel exactly the same, just with a clearer understanding of yourself.

Sometimes the idea of what it means to *be* something can feel extremely overwhelming because we think we need to meet certain expectations, step into a world we're yet to understand and leave behind what we know. And while, yes, some of that might be true, assimilating a queer identity doesn't mean losing yourself: it means gaining more.

Whatever that looks and feels like to *you*.

'I should hide this'

Hiding your sexuality while you figure it out in your mind is common. It's healthy to understand your feelings on your own terms and timeline before communicating it to others. Sometimes when there is too much noise and opinions floating around from third parties it holds us back from doing the internal work we need to do to unpack where we're at, but I would say that isolating yourself entirely isn't the right way to go about things either.

We all need an outlet to express ourselves, even if this takes the form of a close friend or therapist (if your budget allows – though there may also be free services in your country). Keeping secrets (especially if you're like me and value honesty) can make your behaviour, and in turn your entire self, feel deeply inauthentic and misaligned, while also feeding the narrative in your head that all of this is something to be ashamed of, which of course it is not.

If you find yourself slipping into secrecy, just remember that vocalising your thoughts in a *safe* space will help you to process them, and allow you to not get stuck in a grey area of uncertainty (for more on this, *see* chapter 7). Instead, it can help you to find your way through.

'Does this make me look gay?'

Every queer woman knows how overwhelming it can feel trying to decide what to wear, especially when you're in the middle of figuring out your sexuality.

Clothes aren't just fabric: they're intrinsically tied to how we express ourselves and how we feel in our own skin. So if you're reading this and currently standing in your bedroom mirror throwing things on the floor, that's completely normal.

Coming out is like puberty 2.0 and part of that (as much as I wish it wasn't) is doing an audit of your wardrobe and deciding how you want to present yourself to the world. I've personally cycled through eras of crop tops, flannel shirts, sweatpants, all-black outfits, tea dresses and more, before settling on something that feels 'me' (ironically, it's very close to what I started with in the first place).

There's no rush to define your style overnight. It's OK to try things on, both literally and figuratively, and to take the time to see what feels right. Some days you might feel powerful in something bold and expressive, while on other days you may reach for comfort and simplicity. Both are valid.

Give yourself the freedom to experiment, to evolve and, most importantly, to feel at home in whatever you choose to wear. You don't owe the world an explanation or a final version of yourself, but you do owe yourself the freedom to go on that journey.

'I don't want to go down on them, so I can't be into women'

If I could count the number of times I've heard newly out or curious people say this line then I would be rich. It's strange where our brains go immediately when we feel frightened by something alien and new. It's like our inner monologue is screaming, *This is the most out of our comfort zone, unusual thing* ever, *so let's fixate on it, so we can convince ourselves that if we don't know how to do it or we feel* threatened *by it, then we sure as hell should* avoid *it!*

(But in my opinion you shouldn't avoid it, because it's *lots* of fun.)

As humans, we're wired to jump ahead 10 steps when we encounter something new that feels like a threat. Our brains instinctively run through worst-case scenarios to try to protect us, from embarrassment and rejection through to emotional pain or loss. This is part of what psychologists call 'negativity bias' and 'threat-assessment' systems. Certain parts of our brain are highly sensitive to danger cues. In human history, expecting danger was often safer, so these systems were useful. But in today's emotional and social lives, they can misfire, causing us to catastrophise what a certain action, activity or behaviour might mean, or to overestimate just how much judgement or loss we'll face.

This isn't, of course, to say that oral sex will result in rejection, or worse . . . death, but more that the very make-up of our psyche facilitates this 'existential crisis' because it thinks it's doing the right thing to protect us.

There are some instances when this is very useful – for example, that queasy or frightened feeling when we're at a great height or close to a cliff edge – but there are times when it's not so useful, such as when you might actually *want* to jump off the building or cliff, because, say, you'd like to try skydiving or BASE jumping.

I'm not suggesting that *everyone* should love BASE jumping (or in turn going down on someone) but my point is that you can't always trust your fears. Yes, they're there to help keep you safe, but in some scenarios they stop us from having a good time, too!

'Why am I so angry all the time?'

Did you know that anger is actually a secondary emotion?

Beneath it often lies sadness, fear or pain.

In fact, anger usually shows up when those deeper emotions, especially pain, have been pushed down or ignored for too long. And when it comes to sexuality and identity, that emotional mix can be even more complex. Shame, judgement, grief and confusion can all quietly build up in the background, until anger bursts through as the only emotion we feel allowed to express.

I remember the weeks that followed the realisation that I liked women. I moved slower, hung my head in shame and my body physically ached. I had a heavy hurt inside me that as much as I tried, I just couldn't shift.

The smallest things made me angry. The weather, a T-shirt that didn't fit right or the facial expression of a stranger as they glanced across the room. I had zero threshold for anything and I was quick to fly off the handle at others, then immediately feel shame and guilt for it in the aftermath.

When you're at war with yourself, you're also at war with the world. Nothing will ever sit right externally if you can't align internally and that's one of the most painful and hard realisations that you'll have on this journey, because you can't bypass it.

What you can do, though, is look at the root cause of your pain and hurt. Nobody wants to battle themselves or others (and it's certainly not good for our relationships to do that), so it's important to recognise and work through where your reactions are coming from.

Allow yourself to have compassion during this period; working through your sexuality is a *really* hard thing to do and unfortunately there's likely going to be collateral damage along the way. But let's try to minimise that. Learn to communicate your struggles, take a breath and apologise when you need to.

When you don't have an answer for how you're feeling, the world can feel like an incredibly lonely place. It's easy to convince yourself that you're the only one going through it, but that's simply not true.

Let it be known: I was, at times, absolutely an *arsehole* while figuring out my sexuality.

We're all human. And being messy is part of the process.

'Am I losing my reality?'

This is a common thought for many queer women as they enter into a period of questioning and transition, and it all comes down to how much control you perceive yourself to hold, or not to hold.

When we're not grounded in our identity, we feel vulnerable and that vulnerability can make us feel frightened and exposed. It can also often bring up emotions from past situations where we didn't feel in control and vulnerable.

The important thing to do is to ground yourself in the present. Take action on the small things that you can do to be assertive and stay in the driving seat. This could be as simple as maintaining your gym routine, finding a therapist or buying a book you know could help (you can tick that one off your list, because you're reading this).

You don't have to take on the world and come up with all of the answers on day one: it's all about small, consistent steps that will build and maintain your courage and confidence.

You can never *lose* your reality. It might feel blurred but everything in life is temporary – some things just last a little longer than others.

'Has my life up until this point been a lie?'

No time in life is wasted and no periods of our lives are 'fake' or a 'lie'. We show up, behave and experience life through the lens of how we're thinking, feeling and what we know to be true at that moment in time.

Sometimes, though, we gain new knowledge or insight that causes us to reflect on past moments with fresh eyes. We might find ourselves wondering, *If only I had known this then . . .* or *Would I have acted differently?* It's natural to look back and question, but it's important to remember that the choices we made were based on what we knew, felt and understood at the time.

I remember when I was on holiday in Bali in the summer of 2024 and I bought a large papaya from the supermarket (this is going somewhere, I swear). I ate all of it in one sitting, having forgotten to wash the fruit first (something that is recommended, if like me you have a bowel disease) and ended up doubled over in pain for the two days that followed, with Bali belly. When I returned home I spoke to a lot of people about this and they shared how they had always been cautious with fresh fruit and vegetables when travelling to Indonesia, for exactly this reason. I kicked myself, wishing I'd had had that information when I needed it and spared myself rolling around a hotel room bathroom in 30-degree heat, but alas.

That papaya incident taught me something deeper – not just about how to fashion an adult nappy from toilet paper for a three-hour taxi ride back to the airport, but about how we navigate situations with the information we have at the time. I was happy eating my papaya, until my body told me otherwise. It wasn't a mistake or a regret – it was simply something that happened.

When we look past the papaya to the lens of sexuality (a sentence I never thought I'd write), there's really not much difference. Exploring your sexuality is much like choosing to eat some fruit. I'm not saying that it'll cause you to shit yourself – the point is that you can forgive yourself for not having the information that you have now. You weren't living a lie before: you were living within the limits of what you knew – and now you're expanding that.

'What is truly me, and what has been placed upon me?'

This question often arises for queer women when they start to unpack how much of their lives have been shaped by external influences – family, culture, societal norms – rather than their own desires. It's the realisation that maybe some of the things you've pursued, believed in or wanted... weren't entirely motivated by your *own* wants.

We all absorb the opinions and expectations of others, sometimes without even realising it. We make choices based on what seems acceptable, sensible or 'right', but real clarity comes when you start asking: *Do I actually want this? Or have I just been told that I should?*

The only way to answer this honestly is by spending time with yourself. Being alone can feel daunting, especially if you're used to defining yourself through relationships or responsibilities, but solitude holds power. When you strip away the noise and sit with your own thoughts, you begin to hear what's actually yours.

That said, don't isolate yourself completely. We're wired for connection, and community plays a crucial role in feeling safe and supported. But balance is key. You owe it to yourself to turn the volume down on the outside world and tune into the one voice that matters most: your own.

The physical impact of coming out to yourself

We often talk about the *mental* impact of keeping something bottled up, whether that be your sexuality, a secret or just the truth of who you are becoming. But what we don't talk about enough is how much this affects us *physically*. So let's unpack that a bit now:

'Why am I so tired and sick?'

When you're under long-term emotional stress, your body produces more cortisol, a hormone designed to help you cope with short-term threats. But when stress becomes chronic, cortisol can do more harm than good. Too much of it disrupts sleep, impairs digestion, triggers inflammation and undermines your overall sense of well-being.

The stress of hiding your true self, or constantly walking on eggshells around your identity, can show up in your body in strange and distressing ways: insomnia, cold sweats and night-time panic attacks. In more extreme cases, it can even manifest as medical issues that aren't tied to long-term conditions, but are instead symptoms of an overwhelmed nervous system trying to protect you.

So what does this mean? Well, when you suppress big parts of who you are, your body doesn't just shrug it off. It listens. It reacts. It doesn't know whether you're hiding from emotional rejection or a physical predator – your system just knows something isn't safe, and it goes into alert mode.

Understanding this doesn't erase the fear or discomfort, but it can be a relief to know there's a biological reason why it feels so intense. You're not 'too sensitive' or 'overreacting': you're human, and your body is trying to take care of you the best way it knows how.

So what can you do?

The more you can bring peace to your mind, the more your body will begin to relax. They work in tandem – they're not separate entities. Here are some ideas for how you can help yourself:

- **Move your body regularly,** even if it's just a short walk. Movement releases built-up cortisol, produces endorphins and boosts serotonin, the mood-balancing chemical we all need more of during times of stress.
- **Get things out of your head.** Journal, voice-note or speak to someone you trust. Emotional processing helps lighten the cognitive load.
- **Breathe.** I'm not going to tell you to do deep, mindful breathwork, because it's not something I remember to do very often, but if it's in your wheelhouse, go for it! What I do recommend is that you just take a deep breath every so often. It will help bring you back to the present and centre you – trust me.

Above all, give yourself grace. You're not behind. You're becoming, and your body is simply reminding you of how deeply this matters.

Invisible barriers that might stop you from coming out to yourself and others

Sometimes, as much as you want to speak your truth about your identity to yourself and others, there are invisible barriers that hold you back. These internal roadblocks can be deeply rooted, without you even realising they're there.

From internalised homophobia to denial and even emotional paralysis, these experiences can make it incredibly hard to accept yourself, let alone share that truth with anyone else.

In this section, we're going to explore three of the most common things that might be standing in your way, because naming them is often the first step towards moving past them.

1. Internalised homophobia

Shame thrives in the presence of judgement.

Sometimes that judgement comes from the outside, from people who think they know how you *should* live. But often, the harshest voice is the one in your own head.

If you grew up in an environment where being LGBTQ+ was ignored, rejected or outright condemned, it's likely you've absorbed some of those beliefs, whether you're aware of it or not.

One of the most common places these harmful messages can take root is within religious settings. This isn't about criticising religion across the board but it *is* important to recognise the role that certain teachings and environments have played in shaping the experiences of LGBTQ+ individuals.

So how can you shift internalised homophobia?

Sometimes you have to zoom out to see what's really going on. Internalised homophobia can be so deeply embedded that it prevents us from growing into who we truly are. And until we name it for what it is, we can't challenge it.

When your values are shaped by the people you love and respect – family, friends, mentors – it can feel nearly impossible to separate your own voice from theirs. But to live freely, you have to make that distinction: *What do I believe? What's true for me? And what has simply been passed down to me?*

Breaking free means forming your own definitions of right and wrong, and standing firmly in them. That doesn't mean the world around you will change overnight. Some people *will* make you feel ashamed. Some *won't* support your identity. And yes, some of them may leave.

But here's the truth: the people who really matter will meet you on the other side. And the ones who don't? They were never meant to walk the whole way with you.

That's a hard truth to accept, but it's also a liberating one.

2. Denial

'But why not face your feelings?' I hear you ask, and it's a valid question.

When we go through a period of hardship (no matter the size or context) we can either choose to look for the *antidote* to our pain in the people, places or experiences that will heal us, or *mask* those feelings that we're not ready yet to understand or explore.

In the context of sexuality, masking looks different for different people. It could take the form of distracting yourself with drink, sex and substances or it could involve binge/restrictive eating or even throwing yourself obsessively into work with no let-up or time to think.

But why do so many people in denial about their sexuality mask their emotions?

Well ... money, alcohol, drugs, external validation and sex, to name just a few, offer a heady mix of ways to dissociate. They allow us to regain a sense of control or power, block our internal dialogue and feel validated without confronting the pain of emotional intimacy and vulnerability.

Even something as consistent as work can become a convenient escape. It provides an outlet away from our personal lives, where we can pour hours into distracting tasks.

It's easier to blame our sense that everything's 'falling apart' on the stress of an upcoming Q4 marketing report than to face the more confronting truth: that we might be deeply unhappy and out of alignment with our authentic selves.

I wasn't at a place during my late teens/early 20s where I could accept that I had feelings for the same sex. I knew on the surface that something was going on, but the idea of kissing another girl made me feel physically sick with shame.

I needed to maintain control in the situation, because I felt like I was losing it. I convinced myself that it meant *nothing*. Admitting otherwise would mean that I had to face up to the fact that I had feelings for another woman, and that would involve a lot of emotional unpacking that I didn't want to face or do.

I buried the feelings deeply not only because I was frightened of who I was, but also who I would need to *become* to be truly happy. Under the surface I was conscious that I had to change and have hard conversations but I also knew the path wasn't going to be easy, so instead I denied that I needed to go there.

Until I couldn't deny it any more.

So how can you move past denial?

I'm not here to tell you to give up drinking, drugs, sex or whatever other activity you're currently engaging in, because I know how hard these emotions feel, but there comes a time when the lack of wanting to look inside means that our behaviours can affect our health and well-being – and that's a dangerous place to be.

We need to respect our bodies; we need to keep the good people around us close; and we need to, more importantly, respect *ourselves*.

It might take a while to break the habits that keep you masking the emotions, but until you do, you'll live in a never-ending cycle of denial.

3. Emotional paralysis

When you first start to question your sexuality or identity, it can feel like you've been thrown onto an emotional roller coaster you didn't sign up for. One moment you might feel excited, relieved, even – like things are finally clicking into place. And the next you might panic, backtrack or completely shut down. This stop–start cycle can leave you feeling stuck, frozen in uncertainty and unsure which voice in your head to trust.

Analysis paralysis is a state where conflicting thoughts and emotions crash into each other. When you're faced with a lot of uncertainty (about identity, decisions, feelings), your brain tries to overthink every possible outcome. But instead of helping, this overanalysis often leads to not making any decision at all. Over time, this indecision feels safer than acting and possibly being wrong.

Here's the truth: feelings can fluctuate, especially during a period of self-discovery. That doesn't make them any less real. Just because you're unsure doesn't mean you're wrong. Just because it changes shape over time doesn't mean it's not valid. Your identity is allowed to evolve and your confusion is not a failure: it's part of the process.

So how can you move past emotional paralysis?
Here are a few ideas:

- **Give yourself permission to be unsure** – You don't need to have everything figured out right now, or ever. Your identity is yours to define, in your own time.
- **Focus on curiosity, not certainty** – Instead of trying to land on a fixed decision, ask yourself, *What feels most true for me* right now? Let that be enough.
- **Limit comparison** – Other people's journeys are not your benchmark. What worked for someone else may not work for you, and that's OK.

The great thing is that you've already taken a step in reading this book, so the only way from here is up.

To help you feel less alone, I asked my community of queer women to describe what this period of questioning and masking feelings felt like for them, so you can see that you're not the only one experiencing this:

QUEER VOICES

'I dated men furiously to hide it, always struggling to connect and form a meaningful relationship. I occasionally had deep crushes for women and tried (unsuccessfully) to hide it. I would joke with close friends about fancying another woman!'

I hid it in every way that I could ... Internally, it tore me apart every day.

'I hid in every way that I could. To the outside world I lived a typical nuclear family heteronormative lifestyle. Internally, it tore me apart every day.'

'I did everything. Drink, self-harm, avoidance. I spent time alone in my room. Coming to terms with it was difficult – I'll be honest though: I had no idea what I was coming to terms with!'

'I definitely hid behind sleepovers. I started sleeping with women while living with a roommate who definitely just thought I was having more "friends" sleep over than usual. From my family I was able to hide behind my bisexuality, only informing them of the men I dated rather than the women or nonbinary cuties.'

'I grew up in a small conservative town and in the Christian church, where I was told I should pray it away and that being gay was a one-way ticket to hell. At 14 I was outed at school, laughed at, and told by my best friend that the devil had got into me, so I retreated into the closet, dated boys and tried to act straight until sixth form.'

'I would never ever lie if I was directly asked, but I think it's very common for bi people to be assumed to be straight or gay, depending on who they are in a relationship with. There's also – still – a lot of bi phobia and I got bored of having to give receipts and somehow "prove" my bi status, so it became easier not to talk about it very much publicly.'

How to come out to yourself and others (a five-step process)

Now that we've explored some of the main internal blockers that can make it hard to come out, it's time to take a broader view of the journey ahead.

Coming out is a process that often begins with coming out to yourself – an essential and courageous first step. From there, it evolves into deciding if, when and how to share your truth with others.

In the upcoming section, we'll walk through this full journey together, exploring how to navigate each stage with intention, care and safety. You'll learn ways to support your well-being, set boundaries and honour your truth, wherever you are on your path.

Step 1: Coming out to yourself

As we've touched on, coming out to yourself is more than just acknowledging your identity: it's a process of self-discovery, acceptance and growth.

Rather than repeat what we've already covered, I want to share some thoughtful advice from my queer friends, to provide real, lived insights on how they have actioned the ideas in this chapter. The idea is to help you explore your sexuality in a way that feels empowering, grounded and true to *you*, so that you feel confident and ready for whatever comes next. Here's what they have to say:

QUEER VOICES

'Find your queer community. Once I started to attend queer events, making friends along the way, I couldn't imagine ever going back. The queer community is strong, resilient and doesn't take any shit. If they can do it, so can you.'

'Understand that your tastes may change over time. Once you accept that there are no rules restricting your identity, you will feel so free.'

'I joined forums online and confided in a couple of close friends. Take your time. There's no right way.'

'Sexuality coaching, immersing in queer social media and naming the hard things out loud all helped soften any residual negativity I harboured. I also allowed myself to validate and feel all of my emotions through meditation.'

> **The queer community is strong, resilient and doesn't take any shit. If they can do it, so can you.**

'Coming out gradually increased my confidence. Each time I had a positive experience sharing my queer identity with someone else, it made it easier the next time.'

'When I gave myself permission and accepted that I was gay, I never looked back or thought about going back in the closet. Because I'm straight-passing, I still deal with coming out almost every day to a co-worker or a doctor or other people I come into contact with, but that's getting easier.'

Step 2: How to know when it feels right to 'come out' to others

Everyone arrives at making decisions differently: some people sit on things and analyse the options and others arrive at what feels right sporadically.

My advice is to trust your instincts and tune in to your intuition. When you think about coming out to others, does the idea feel freeing or does it spark unease? There's a big difference between feeling nervous (because doing something new or vulnerable is naturally scary) and sensing that now simply isn't the right time, because it could put your livelihood or safety in danger.

An unsafe situation might look like living with someone who is emotionally unpredictable, being financially dependent on people who might not react well, or knowing in your gut that disclosing your truth could genuinely put your well-being at risk. If any of this resonates with your circumstances, it doesn't make your identity or experience any less real or valid, it just means safety comes first, and you need to prioritise that.

That said, keeping major parts of yourself hidden for too long can take a real emotional toll. The longer you suppress who you are, the heavier that burden becomes. That's why it's so important to have a plan, one that takes into account different possible outcomes and how you'll handle them.

A helpful way to start is by imagining how you *might* feel after taking that step. Will you feel lighter, relieved, more grounded? Or perhaps anxious, uncertain or even regretful? Visualising these emotional outcomes can bring clarity and give you a greater sense of control.

The more prepared you feel, the more confident you'll be in choosing *when* and *how* to share your truth.

No two coming-out experiences are the same, but I believe that by hearing someone else's truth, we can sometimes feel a little more connected to our own. So, I asked my queer community to share their experiences:

QUEER VOICES

'Some friends and family felt sad that I hadn't felt safe to tell them earlier in life and wondered why I hadn't trusted them with that information. But ultimately those conversations, although hard, made our relationships stronger.'

'While my mother always knew I was queer, I didn't officially come out to my parents until I was 17. My father responded by telling me that he didn't want to look at my face. He avoided me for three days, not speaking a word to me. He mellowed out eventually, but I was so shocked by him. My advice for coming out? Never assume how it will go!'

My advice for coming out? Never assume how it will go!

'I was outed several times before I was ready. That was largely because my presentation was not particularly heteronormative. Weirdly, it helped, as it made me realise that people actually don't give a f*ck (in a nice way).'

'I had a good coming-out process. The first thing my stepmom said when I came out was, "I understand – you love hearts not parts."'

'When I came out, my mum tried to tell me about her own "close female friendships" and that she might've been a lesbian in a different era. Thinking back, this was quite cool of my mum. But, as a teenager, this just seemed cringe.'

'Being outed was humiliating, but it taught me resilience. My advice: their rejection says nothing about your worth and more about the limits of their world and capacity for empathy – hold on for the people who meet you with love.'

'One friend (who is now an awesome ally) responded when I came out to her as bi with, "Oh god, you're not going to become one of those people who make being gay their whole personality are you?" I said I wasn't planning on putting it on my voicemail message but I was looking forward to no longer pretending I'm straight.'

Step 3: Complications if you're already in a relationship or marriage

A lot of the personal messages I receive online are from women looking for advice on how to navigate romantic feelings for other women that have come up for them while they're in long-term relationships with or (more often) marriages to men.

The messages are often fraught with worry as they desperately grapple to explain that they think they might like women, knowing they need to do something about it, yet having no clue where to begin.

Really my advice to women who feel this way is the same as in steps 1 and 2. You need to get really clear on how you feel about this new attraction and understand where it's coming from, what it's trying to tell you and what you'd like to do about it.

For some women in relationships, simply acknowledging and sharing these feelings with their partner might feel like enough, without any immediate urge to act on them.

But in many cases, especially where there's a history of repression – such as a lack of intimacy, a longing to rediscover yourself or a deep pull to explore a part of you that's gone untouched – I've found that most women *do* eventually feel the desire to act on those feelings, even if they can't admit it right away.

The real challenge, then, becomes how to navigate that conversation with your partner.

There's a difference between 'loving' someone and being 'in love' with someone and often this is the first question you need to sit down and really unpack (as terrifying and awful as it sounds). Sometimes we can wander through life on autopilot, never stopping to really ask ourselves if the life we're living is making us truly happy, and getting real and honest about this is going to form the basis of how you come out to your partner, whether you move forwards with them or without them.

If you've decided you would like to explore this part of you, but you don't want to leave your partnership, then this is a conversation you need to have. Both of you need to discuss whether it is something you would be open to exploring (either solo or together as a pair). It's a hard conversation to have, but they deserve to know the truth about the person they're in a partnership with, regardless of the outcome.

To start the conversation you could introduce the idea by discussing a podcast or article that you've read around the idea of open relationships, to gauge their reaction, or you could go straight in and explain that you've been feeling a certain way for a while and wanted to let them in, because it didn't feel right not to talk about it.

The main thing to remember is to hold respect for your partner and assure them that it doesn't change anything about your dynamic. It's purely an expansion of the relationship and something that you'd like for both of you to navigate together, because you value what you have.

On the flip side, if, after deep reflection, you've come to the difficult decision that this is a journey you need to take *without* your partner, then it's fair to say, this *will* be one of the hardest conversations you'll have.

There's no easy way to say it, but being honest, as painful as it may be in the moment, is ultimately the kinder path for both of you. Staying in a relationship that no longer has a future only prolongs the hurt for everyone involved.

Of course there are many things to consider if you've been with this person for a long time. Perhaps children, pets and family members are in the mix in addition to finances, property and material belongings. None of this is easy and even if you've come to the conclusion that the relationship no longer serves you, it doesn't mean that you don't still have an emotional bond with this person.

If you find yourself in this situation, then I really feel for you, but I also have faith that you've got this. It takes a lot of courage to choose honesty in a situation where you could so easily continue in silence. But at the end of the day, if you want to create a life of true happiness and authenticity, it involves losing some things and people along the way to make room for the new.

And that loss may only be temporary. I know plenty of women who have redefined their relationships yet still have the presence of their ex-partners in their lives, too. As hard as it can be in the moment, everyone will ultimately be happier when the truth is out, so it is helpful to remember that.

Let's hear now how some of the queer women in my community handled these sorts of situations:

QUEER VOICES

'When I came out to my ex-husband after five years of being married, he affirmed my queer identity and didn't fetishise or objectify my attraction to other women. I think it helped that my coming out didn't change anything about our relationship status: I wanted to remain monogamous. Thankfully, I was married to someone that was already an ally to the LGBTQ+ community, so I didn't have to do any extra education or coaching about how he could support me. While he and I ultimately divorced several years later (and I'm currently engaged to a woman!), I'm glad the dissolution of our relationship had nothing to do with issues over my queer identity.'

'One of my only regrets about coming out is that I was in a long-term relationship with a man. I wish I'd not tied up someone else's emotions as collateral damage. I've come to forgive myself now as I genuinely didn't know a better way of navigating the complex feelings at the time. If I could offer any advice to others on this, it would be to lead with honesty and compassion for all parties involved and affected.'

'There is no easy way out but through. You have to be honest. Some like to rip the bandage off and tell their spouse and kids all at once, while others choose to do it separately. It's imperative to know your unique situation first.'

'It was heartbreaking to end my 12-year relationship with my boyfriend. It still bothers me now, but I know he's moved on – he's happy that I'm happy, and he knows I never meant to hurt him. Whether you're in a relationship with the wrong person because you're closeted or you're not aligned in other ways, it will always catch up with you, so you might as well be honest.'

'My kids were amazing! I told them in the context of them talking to me about their conversations in their schools during Pride Month, explaining that I am bi and what that means to me. They were so open-minded, so it felt very natural. I just made sure they had space for loads of questions, both at that moment and later on.'

There is no easy way out but through. You have to be honest.

'For me, when I came out to my ex-partner, it was quite a spur-of-the-moment thing. I knew I wanted to come out to him, but I didn't plan it. I ended up telling him on one of our dates. I think this was the best thing I could have done because I didn't feel an immense build-up and it felt more natural, which took my own internal pressure off.'

Step 4: Choosing who to tell

Embarking on a journey that's reflective, joyful, painful, confusing and challenging, whether it's about your sexuality, gender or a major life decision, is already a lot to carry. What can make it even trickier, though, is if people tag along uninvited, offering their opinions and inserting themselves into something that was never theirs to navigate.

These people could be well-meaning family members, friends, colleagues or anyone else you've shared your feelings with in a bid to get clarity. But the problem with this (other than having to keep updating everyone on your latest thoughts and feelings like a sort of rolling broadcast) is that it can all feel a bit *much*, especially at the start of your journey, when you're likely still piecing things together as you go along.

That's why it's so important to remember you don't have to tell everyone everything all at once.

Think of it as a layered approach. Begin with the people closest to you – the ones you trust, who've consistently had your back, or who you may have already confided in, even a little. Then, when it feels right, you can move outwards to the next circle – those who aren't quite as close but still play a meaningful role in your life and who you feel should be part of this chapter.

This isn't about rushing. It's about moving at your own pace and deciding who gets access to this part of you, when and how it feels right.

Don't make your choices based on who you think *should* know; focus instead on who you *want* to share it with. That way, your decision is rooted in intention, not obligation.

Christmas cards

An analogy I like to use to describe how it feels to come out is writing Christmas cards. It's less of a thing now that we all live online, but back in the 1990s my parents would spend entire evenings writing out Christmas cards to people who they hadn't seen all year, updating them about their life, where they'd moved to, how I was doing in school and what plans my dad had for the garden (spoiler: it was always creating some kind of decking area, so I think people were poised for that specific update).

The point that I'm trying to make here is that I thought I needed to approach telling people about my newfound sense of self like writing out Christmas cards to anyone I'd ever encountered, updating them on the news. That way, if we did see each other they'd be prepared and up-to-date, and there would be no awkwardness between us.

However, what I quickly realised is that putting other people's feelings and potential awkwardness about a piece of information before my own needs serves little purpose. People will react in the way they want to and it's not my responsibility to make them feel a certain type of way.

I also think that letting people into your life should be a privilege, so I switched the idea of writing 'Christmas cards' to writing 'party invites'. If I like you enough and you're a hoot, then you can come and join me and the rest of my mates in the VIP area where we're not just broadcasting but *celebrating*.

Step 5: Coming out is continuous (not just a one-time thing)

There are of course times when (in contrast to the advice above) it might feel like you need to share parts of yourself in a bid to clarify or clear things up with others. This is totally valid, so long as (again) it's coming from *you* and doesn't feel forced.

There have been plenty of times at work, when meeting new people or on dates when people assume my sexuality and identity and out of principle (even though it's annoying to have to start the conversation) I've corrected them. I don't do this all the time and it really depends on how much I value the connection/if I will be seeing them again, but most of the time I see it as an educational opportunity that I'm pleased to pick up. I do recognise, though, that not everyone is afforded that luxury and sometimes staying quiet can protect your peace and safety. Whichever approach you take is valid.

Coming out, regardless of whether you like to yap on like me or not, is going to be a continuous process. This is mainly because society is programmed to think that everyone is straight and even though we're getting better at not assuming, the bias will always be there in our subconscious. (I do it myself at times; we all do.)

There is no specific way to get comfortable with this, other than time. The more confident you feel in yourself, the easier it is to let other people's assumptions roll off you, whether you choose to correct them or not.

> ### Coming out can bring you closer to other people
>
> I lived above my 70-year-old landlord for five years when I first moved to London and only a few months before I moved out did he clock on to the fact that I dated women. It wasn't a conscious choice not to share this fact with him – the subject just simply never came up.
>
> He found out during Pride Month (the conversation had been around him needing help with something, and me planning on being unavailable due to being covered head to toe in glitter and mainlining a lot of tequila) and he, to my surprise, reacted by being quite *moved* by the information (the coming out; not the tequila).
>
> A few days later I came home to find an envelope full of newspaper clippings on my front doorstep. It was a selection of articles around

> prominent queer women in the media, with a note attached that read: 'I thought of you and thought you might like to read these.'
>
> I still have the clippings today. They remind me that there is so much goodness in the world if you choose to share, regardless of what generation someone belongs to.
>
> Coming out continuously over time doesn't have to be a bad thing; being vulnerable can bring you closer to people regardless of the subject.
>
> We would all do well to remember that.

The good news is that there are countless coming-out stories out there, shared through social media, podcasts, books and documentaries, which you can explore at your own pace. These stories matter. They highlight the many different ways people find their truth, and I encourage you to seek them out. They're powerful reminders that there's no single 'right' way to step into who you are.

But since we're on the subject of vulnerability, I think it's time I share my own coming-out story with you.

MY STORY

Back in 2012 I was walking home from work. It was late summer and the sun was setting over the hill in South East London that I was temporarily calling home with my aunt and uncle.

I'd been in the city for around three months and had been talking to (but never meeting up with) girls. After 'Barbie-Gate with Becky', I'd started to accept that I might be more curious about my sexuality than I'd let myself admit. So, one evening, I set up a Tinder profile and let my finger 'accidentally' slide my preferences to 'women'. I was fully intending to change it back, but when I saw photos of girls with charcuterie boards, offering up cosy film nights and walks with their puppies I quite quickly decided that it sounded much nicer than what was on offer from the men.

I dialled my parents' home number as I usually did every couple of days to check in with my mum. I had no plans for our conversation to be anything other than explaining how my day had been, listening to her day and then going home to have a nice meal with my aunt and uncle, but I guess the setting and timing of this particular phone call that night lent itself to the conversation being something more.

'You know Johnny* has moved to London now?!' my mum explained, with an excited undertone.

Johnny was a very clever guy who had an interest in history and politics and was wasted at his part-time job at the local coffee shop near my parents' house. We had been on one date when I was in college, during which we'd met for a steak, he'd tried to kiss me in my mum's Fiesta, which I was driving at the time, I'd panicked, refused and driven off into the distance with the tyres screeching, and we'd never spoken again.

'Right,' I said flatly. 'Good for him.'

'He's a nice guy, you know,' she said back, not dropping the subject.

'I'm sure he is –' I paused – 'but I have no interest in dating guys.'

[silence]

'I want to date girls.'

[more prolonged silence]

I stopped dead in the road and realised what I'd done.

'I'll call you back.'

After a minute, just long enough for my heart to stop trying to escape my chest, fear started to morph into something hotter. Rage. What began as a worry that my mother wouldn't understand me, that she might judge or dismiss everything I'd been working through, twisted into anger that she hadn't said *anything* at all. Why didn't she jump in to congratulate me on finally naming this part of myself? Why didn't she ask even one question, the way I'd spent months interrogating my own feelings?

What I failed to recognise, though, was that it was a Tuesday evening in mid-September, and she had one hand in the oven making my dad a quiche and a phone in the other, while I was communicating an existential crisis of identity – one that, if I'm totally honest, I was still in the midst of figuring out myself.

I learned that night that timing really is *everything* when you're wanting to have a deep and meaningful conversation with someone, and it's not something I'm very good at.

My mother didn't speak to me for a few days after I dropped the news (which I later elaborated on in a text message confirming that I was bisexual and 'excited to open up my options'). The continued non-response enraged me even more.

I rang the house phone a few times only to be greeted by my dad saying that she apparently needed time to come to terms with what I'd said. He, on the other hand, was very upset about the fact that I hadn't had a chance to return his Dido CD in the post and was concerned that his alphabetisation of music in the living room bookshelf was going to crumble to the ground if I didn't 'hotfoot' it to the post office.

My dad didn't care one jot about the news – not in a neglectful way but in an entirely unfazed, 'what has this got to do with anything' way. Which I appreciated and needed more than anything at that moment.

But after around a week of awkward silence, he decided enough was enough and a conversation took place between him and my mother, which I've never been privy to.

I don't want to ask what was discussed between the two of them, but all I know is that she miraculously turned herself around and became what I am proud to say is one of the most supportive and caring allies, holding space for not just conversations about my own sexuality, but for the understanding of *others* too.

I'd always wondered what went through her head during that period, though, and around seven years after that night, curiosity got the better of me.

I set up a podcast microphone on the coffee table of their house and asked her if she would record an episode about 'coming out' with me. She agreed to share, because she hoped recording a piece of content from the perspective of a parent in this process might help others to grow and learn from her experience.

I thought interviewing my mother for a piece of very personal social media content might be a mistake. I was worried she wouldn't know what to say, or even worse, not be able to handle it, but I'm proud to say that those 30 minutes with her were not only a privilege to experience, but something that brought us closer together and healed the uncertainty that I didn't know was still lingering inside me, years on.

I'll summarise what she shared in that conversation:

- She told me she felt guilty for not realising I'd been struggling with my sexuality long before I was able to open up about it.
- She admitted she was scared: of the abuse I might face, and of what my life could look like. She didn't know anyone in the LGBTQ+ community, and like me when I first came out, her understanding was limited, shaped only by the media and her own experiences.
- She also said she had to let go of the expectations she'd privately built for my future.
- She acknowledged that those hopes were based more on *her* desires than mine, and with time, she saw that clinging to them was, in some ways, selfish.
- And perhaps most vulnerably, she admitted she was afraid I would change, and in turn that the close relationship we had would change too.

Knowing her as well as I do, I believe this last point was her biggest fear. At the heart of it, she was terrified of losing me. The idea that I was stepping into a world she didn't understand made her worry I might be stepping away from her too.

It reminded me that people's first reactions, especially to big, life-changing news, are often less about *you*, and more about *them* – where they're at emotionally, what they fear and the insecurities they carry.

But with time, those reactions can change.

This isn't to excuse judgement from parents, friends, colleagues or anyone else you might encounter on your coming-out journey, but more to say that allowing someone a moment of grace is a kind of patience that we would do well to practise (even if it feels frustrating at the time!).

Of course, if someone ultimately cannot meet you with the kindness or respect you deserve, you have every right to reconsider whether that relationship still has a place in your life. But just as you've extended understanding and compassion to yourself throughout this process, it can be worth offering others the same chance to reflect and grow.

I explained this recently to a friend as being like cracking open an Easter egg. Often the first crack is resilience (a reactionary response) and the second (or third, fourth, fifth) crack is the break, where the emotions and true feelings finally come out.

I'm proud of my mum – and also my dad, for giving her the additional crack that she needed in order to open up her Easter egg.

Final thoughts

My biggest value in life is honesty and keeping something so big and important from the people I loved so much – my parents – always felt wrong, yet I don't regret my choices.

Yes, my timing could've been better, but I also recognise how frustrated and misaligned to that value of honesty I felt and getting it out of my system was the one thing I knew I needed to do in order to move forwards.

With integrity, you always run the risk of losing what you love – but being honest about who you are is a choice. And personally, I would always rather risk losing something or someone, and making way for the truth, than keeping it secret.

That being said, there have only ever been two moments in my 32 years of living when I have *genuinely* feared losing the love of my mother. One was when I read a text message saying that she'd had a stroke and had been taken to hospital and the other was the night that I came out.

It made me realise that perhaps it is not being seen for who we truly are that we fear the most, but the idea of losing all that we hold close instead.

COMING OUT

The number one question that goes through every queer person's mind in the seconds before they come out or share their true identity with someone that they care deeply for is simply this:

'Will you still love me when you know the truth?'

At its core, coming out is about wanting to be seen, to be truly accepted for who you are and who you're becoming, to have someone sit beside you, listen without judgement, put their own fears aside, and meet you with care and curiosity.

This is what acceptance looks like.

I used to wonder how powerful it would be if everyone had the tools to navigate coming out with kindness, respect and compassion – for themselves and for others – and now they do.

It's a privilege for someone to know who you *really* are; remember that.

TWO

Labels

Technically I have what doctors would describe as a 'tumour' in my brain. It's benign but for a very long time I felt exhausted, fatigued and struggled to complete the most basic of tasks without feeling like I was trudging through mud.

Over the course of one very long and tiring summer I found myself bounced around different hospitals for various brain scans (which mainly involved me being packed into an MRI machine like a little sandwich in a lunch box) and asked to lie still for 45 minutes at a time, to figure out what was going on.

Eventually they discovered that I had a small growth, which was causing the chemicals in my body to be completely out of balance. I was put on medication to bring everything back to a normal state, and to stop the growth from, well... growing.

You're probably wondering what this story has to do with sexuality and labels? As much as I'd love to claim that my altered brain chemistry has somehow turned me into a 'supercharged gay', that's not quite it.

I'm sharing this story to illustrate how people react when I (albeit rarely) reveal this new piece of information to them.

Most people don't know how to process it. I watch their faces shift into confusion the moment they hear the word 'tumour', as if they're trying to figure out whether I'm about to drop dead mid-conversation or live to see another day.

They get stuck on the 'headline' version of the story because it doesn't fit neatly into a box. It's unfamiliar, and their curiosity often spills out in awkward questions as they try to make sense of something they've never encountered before, yet want to understand.

There's a deep need in them to find an explanation, to label it, tidy it up and move on. But they can't, and we are left staring at each other until I fill the silence with a joke to put an end to it all.

This is the exact way I feel about discussing my sexuality.

Confused?

Let me help.

An introduction to labels

There's something about the human brain that craves certainty, simplicity and structure. We like things to make sense. We want stories to follow a clear arc and people to come with definitions. So when something doesn't sit neatly in a box, or worse, when it resists the box altogether, it makes others uncomfortable. And more often than not, it can make *us* uncomfortable too.

This is one of the many reasons I've decided to write a chapter on labels.

Labels can be incredibly helpful and powerful. They can give us language for things we've felt but never been able to articulate. They can connect us to communities, affirm our place in the world and offer a sense of identity that makes us feel more at home in ourselves. But they can also feel confusing, restricting or premature, especially when we're still figuring things out.

In this chapter, we're going to unpack:

- Why we use labels
- How to pick a label (or decide *not* to use one)
- What common labels mean now, and how to make sense of them for *you*
- Whether they're necessary, and under what conditions they help or hurt

- How labels can shift with time, experience and changing of self-understanding – and that it's OK to change your mind

Whether you're someone who finds comfort in clear definitions or who feels boxed in by them, this chapter is for you. My goal isn't to push you towards any specific label, but to offer you the language, understanding and space to consider what *feels right for you*, now, and as you continue to grow.

Because at the end of the day, what matters most is whether the label, or lack of a label, feels honest and freeing for you, not whether it matches someone else's expectation or definition.

Why do we feel the need to use labels?

Putting a label on your identity based on who you like to kiss and/or sleep with, and then broadcasting it to the world is, when you stop and think about it, kind of a strange concept. Yet it's something many of us do, often without questioning it.

Why we do it partly lies in how we're wired. Humans are built for meaning. From an early age we learn to categorise, sort and name everything around us: people, behaviours, emotions, experiences. This isn't just a habit – it's how our brains create a sense of safety and predictability in an otherwise complex and uncertain world.

Labels help us make sense of ourselves and others. They provide structure where there might otherwise be confusion and offer a sense of control when everything feels in flux.

When it comes to sexuality, labels function like signposts: they give language to our internal experiences and offer a pathway towards connection and belonging. For many people, identifying with a term like lesbian, bisexual, pansexual or queer can ease the tension between what they feel on the inside and how they show up in the world. Labels provide clarity, reduce anxiety and allow us to communicate something that might otherwise take paragraphs to explain.

This is part of why the Kinsey Scale made such an impact when it was introduced in 1948 by American biologist and sexologist Alfred Kinsey. His research proposed that sexuality isn't binary but exists on a sliding scale from 0 (exclusively heterosexual) to 6 (exclusively homosexual), with many people falling somewhere in between. It was one of the first mainstream attempts to visualise sexual orientation as a continuum, and his work helped challenge the rigid categories of the time.

Over the years, Kinsey's scale became part of pop culture, with TV stars and Hollywood actors referring to themselves as numbers on the scale: a 'Kinsey 3' or 'Kinsey 5'. Today, it's often referenced more conceptually than literally, but it still serves as a reminder that most of us don't fit neatly at either end of a binary. Our experiences are more fluid, more complex and much more personal.

So if we collectively accept that sexuality exists on a spectrum, why do we still feel the need to *label* it?

The short answer: because labels offer comfort and belonging.

However, they also come with pressure and limitations. Sometimes choosing a label isn't just about what feels right personally, it also means navigating the societal or political weight that certain words carry. For example, terms like lesbian or queer can feel empowering to some but loaded or even alienating to others depending on cultural, generational or community context.

This complexity plays a role in why a study of sexual and gender minority youth found that about 'one in three now use "nontraditional labels, such as pansexual, queer, or genderfluid" rather than more widely recognised terms like "gay" or "straight".' This suggests that many young people are looking for words that match the *full nuance* of their experiences, rather than fitting themselves into a box that doesn't quite feel right.

And yet, not everyone wants to use a label at all, and that's valid too.

While our brains are wired to categorise, we're also wired to *resist* being boxed in when it threatens our sense of authenticity. For some people, refusing a label can be a way to preserve openness, to protect themselves from judgement or to avoid the pressure to perform an identity that doesn't feel settled. Psychologically, not choosing a label can serve as a kind of boundary, a way to create space for fluidity, exploration and autonomy.

Choosing (or not choosing) a label is a deeply personal decision. It may feel affirming for one person and restricting for another. Some people pick a label, live with it for years and later change it. Others prefer something intentionally vague or decide not to name their identity at all.

There's no right or wrong way to navigate this.

> ## Who is the label for, anyway?
>
> Although labels are comforting for many people, and leaning into them can bring a deeper sense of belonging in your identity, we do have to stop and wonder *who* they are actually made for. Is it for us, to bring us a sense of self? Or is it for other people's benefit, so they can understand how to treat us based on the usually limited knowledge they have of what the particular wording actually means?
>
> (There's no right answer to this, by the way – it's purely a prompt for you to consider as you read through this chapter.)

How to pick a label

Everyone makes it sound so simple. Have a little think about what you like and don't like, select from a small, pre-existing list of labels that might fit the bill, slap one on yourself and then carry on with your life... Oh, and be prepared to bat away all of the questions and judgements from other people once you have.

What often happens – in my personal experience and from what I've heard from friends and my online community – is closer to this trajectory:

1. Panic.
2. Question what's going on with your sexuality for an indefinite period of time (this may include some denial, wine, podcasts, existential crisis, questionable decisions, etc. – as discussed in chapter 1).
3. Finally accept that you want to find a new way to identify.
4. Have a look at a pre-existing list of labels to find the one closest to how you feel.
5. Pick one (sometimes you'll be happy with your choice; other times you'll still feel confused).
6. Tell people what you've picked like a public service announcement.

7. Continue living your life and perhaps using the label if people prod you on it.
8. Have an experience or something happen to you that makes you question that label.
9. Panic again.
10. Go back to drinking wine and engaging in questionable life choices.
11. Stick with what you've chosen or redefine it again by choosing another label.
12. Repeat the cycle.

Labels are a controversial topic. A lot of people, as I mentioned above, find comfort in defining themselves by a certain identity, but others struggle with labels either because they can't find the correct one to match how they feel for their situation, or simply because they don't want to be boxed in.

And when it comes to labels, the list is ever-growing. For some people this offers more of an opportunity to find something they align with, but for others it can sometimes feel overwhelming.

Talk to others

It's validating to hear stories of how others choose to label or not label their sexualities. Social media, podcasts and books are a great way to hear these stories and work through your own journey at your own pace.

If you feel comfortable then you can also communicate with others about how you're feeling. Sometimes speaking things out loud can help you to process better and also make the situation less serious and scary.

Hearing how others view their sexualities has been crucial to me accepting my own. What can feel like a really daunting time can be made much lighter by hearing that you're not alone and also receiving the encouragement of others who know you well, to ground you and normalise your racing thoughts.

What are the labels?

There are not only labels for our sexual identity, but the world also offers ready-made categories for gender, gender identity, relationship styles and more. We're handed a kind of 'set menu' of identities: options that are widely accepted, familiar and easy for most people to understand. It's a one-size-fits-all approach. Predictable, controlled and often seen as the 'safe' route.

But in my opinion, what we really need is more of an à la carte menu – something that allows us to mix, match and customise our identities to reflect who we truly are. After all, identity isn't fixed. It should be flexible, personal and made to fit *you*.

I'd like to share some of these terms with you below. While this isn't a complete list (since language and terminology are always evolving; for the latest definitions, check out glaad.org/reference/terms/), it offers a general overview of commonly used phrases and identity markers that describe different preferences and ways people express who they are. As you read through you might find that your identity becomes clearer for you or you might find that you don't want to align with a label. There is no 'correct' way to do this, but I would encourage you to keep your mind open.

Sexuality

Straight – Otherwise known as a heterosexual, meaning they are romantically and/or sexually attracted to people of the opposite gender.

Gay – A person who is romantically and/or sexually attracted to people of the same gender. Most commonly, 'gay' refers to men who are attracted to other men, but it can also be used more broadly as an umbrella term for anyone who is same-gender attracted, including women.

Lesbian – Refers to a woman who is romantically and/or sexually attracted to other women. It is a specific type of homosexual orientation and is generally used to describe women who identify as female and are exclusively or primarily attracted to other women.

Sapphic – Referring to women who are attracted to other women. The term comes from **Sappho**, an ancient Greek poet from the island of Lesbos, whose poetry often expressed desire and love between women. In contemporary usage, it broadly encompasses romantic or sexual attraction between women or femme-presenting individuals. It's often used in phrases like 'sapphic love' and 'sapphic relationships', and can include lesbians, bisexual women, queer women, and others who identify with attraction to women.

Bisexual – A person who is romantically and/or sexually attracted to more than one gender, typically to both men and women, though not necessarily in the same way or to the same degree. Bisexuality does not require equal attraction to all genders, and it does not imply being attracted to only two genders: many bisexual people are also attracted to nonbinary individuals.

Pansexual – Someone who is romantically and/or sexually attracted to people regardless of their gender identity or biological sex. Pansexual people may feel attraction to men, women, nonbinary individuals and people of all gender identities. The prefix 'pan-' means 'all', reflecting the idea that gender is not a determining factor in their attraction. Pansexuality is distinct but related to bisexuality: both involve attraction to multiple genders, but pansexuality emphasises inclusivity of all gender identities.

Asexual – Refers to someone who experiences little or no sexual attraction to others. Asexuality is a spectrum, meaning that asexual people may have a range of experiences: some may feel no sexual attraction at all, while others might experience it rarely, or only under specific circumstances (such as within a strong emotional bond). Asexuality is about sexual attraction, not necessarily romantic attraction: some asexual people are still romantically attracted to others and may identify as heteroromantic, homoromantic, biromantic, etc.

Aromantic – Someone who experiences little or no romantic attraction to others. Aromantic people may not desire romantic relationships or may not experience feelings like 'falling in love' in the way that romantic people do. Like asexuality, aromanticism exists on a spectrum: some aromantic individuals might feel romantic attraction rarely, or only under specific conditions. It's important to note that being aromantic is about romantic attraction, not sexual attraction. An aromantic person can have any sexual orientation: they might be asexual, bisexual, straight, gay, etc.

Demisexual – Someone who only experiences sexual attraction after forming a strong emotional bond with another person. Demisexual people do not usually feel sexual attraction based on appearance or initial encounters. The emotional connection required is often deep and personal, but it doesn't always have to be romantic. Demisexuality is considered part of the asexual spectrum because it involves experiencing sexual attraction less frequently or under specific conditions compared to non-sexual people.

Queer – 'Queer' as a sexual identity is a broad and inclusive term used by people who do not identify as exclusively heterosexual and/or cisgender. It can refer to a wide range of sexual orientations, gender identities, or both. Some people use queer because more specific labels (like gay, bisexual, pansexual, etc.) don't fully capture their experience. Others choose it as a political or cultural identity – and use a capital letter: 'Queer' – emphasising a rejection of traditional norms around sexuality and gender. Historically, queer was used as a slur, but it has been reclaimed by many within the LGBTQ+ community.

Fluid – Often referred to as sexual fluidity, 'fluid' describes someone whose sexual orientation or attraction can change over time. A fluid person might experience shifts in who they are attracted to, such as being more attracted to one gender at one point in life, and another later on. These changes can happen over time, in different contexts or without a clear pattern. 'Fluid' is often used by people who don't feel fixed or limited to one specific label like gay, straight or bisexual. It reflects a flexible and evolving sense of identity.

Gender

Male – 'Male' as a gender identity refers to a person who identifies as a man or boy, typically aligning with cultural and social roles associated with masculinity. This identity can be based on biological sex assigned at birth, but not always: some people assigned female at birth may identify as male (transgender men). Being male as a gender identity is about how a person internally understands and experiences their own gender, rather than just physical characteristics. In summary, male is a gender identity that encompasses those who see themselves as men, regardless of their sex assigned at birth.

Female – 'Female' as a gender identity refers to a person who identifies as a woman or girl, typically aligning with cultural and social roles associated with femininity. This identity may or may not correspond with the sex assigned at birth: some people assigned male at birth may identify as female (transgender women). Being female as a gender identity is about how someone personally understands and experiences their own gender, beyond just physical or biological traits. In short, female is a gender identity that includes those who see themselves as women, regardless of their assigned sex at birth.

Cisgender – The term 'cisgender' refers to a person whose gender identity matches the sex they were assigned at birth. For example, someone who was assigned female at birth and identifies as a woman is cisgender.

Nonbinary – The term 'nonbinary' refers to a gender identity for people who do not exclusively identify as either male or female. Nonbinary individuals may feel their gender is somewhere in between, a mix of both, neither, or outside the traditional categories of man and woman. This identity can include a wide variety of experiences and labels, such as genderqueer, genderfluid, agender, and more. Nonbinary is part of the broader gender diversity spectrum and challenges the idea that there are only two fixed genders.

Transgender – Transgender (often shortened to 'trans') is an umbrella term for people whose gender identity differs from the sex they were assigned at birth. For example, someone assigned male at birth who identifies as a woman, or someone assigned female at birth who identifies as a man, is transgender. Being transgender is about a person's internal sense of gender, not their physical characteristics or medical history. Not all transgender people undergo medical transition (like hormone therapy or surgery), and that's completely valid.

Agender – This refers to a gender identity where a person does not identify with any gender or feels neutral or absent of gender altogether. People who identify as agender may see themselves as having no gender or as being genderless. Agender individuals might also use terms like gender-neutral or genderless to describe their experience.

Intersex – A person who is born with biological sex characteristics (such as chromosomes, hormones, gonads or genitalia) that don't fit typical definitions of male or female. This can include variations in chromosomes (like XXY or XYY), hormone levels or physical anatomy.

Intersex is about biological traits, not gender identity or sexual orientation: intersex people can identify as male, female, nonbinary or any gender. Being intersex is a natural variation in human biology and is not the same as transgender.

Relationship structures

Monogamy – A relationship structure where a person has one romantic or sexual partner at a time.

Polyamory – Having multiple consensual romantic and/or sexual relationships at the same time, with the knowledge and consent of everyone involved.

Open relationship or ethical non-monogamy – A committed relationship where partners agree that they may have sexual or romantic encounters outside the primary relationship, often without those outside partners being considered 'primary'.

Swinging – Couples consensually engaging in sexual activities with others, often in social or party settings, but usually maintaining an emotional primary partnership.

Triad/throuple – A three-person romantic and/or sexual relationship where all partners are involved with each other.

Polygamy – Being married to more than one spouse at the same time, often associated with specific cultural or religious contexts.

It's a lot to take in, isn't it? Like learning a completely different language and everyone else seems to already know the rules. Feeling overwhelmed is totally normal – you're not alone.

But instead of throwing more terms and definitions at you, I want to pause and share a bit of my own journey in understanding my identity. Sometimes hearing how someone else navigated their path with labels can make things feel a lot more digestible and a little less confusing. Along the way, you'll also hear from others about how they've chosen, or decided not to choose, labels that fit them, showing just how personal and varied this process can be.

My path wasn't linear, and I definitely didn't wake up one day with all the answers. It was a process of exploration, reflection and learning to trust myself. Hopefully, by sharing it, I can help shed some light on the parts that might still feel unclear for you right now.

LABELS

MY STORY

Everyone now knows that I like kissing women, but there was also a time when I liked kissing men and the journey to understanding my sexuality hasn't been a straightforward one.

When I first came out in 2015 I identified as bisexual, but after only a few months of dating women, the label didn't feel right. I was attracted to women in a way that I didn't feel with men and that confused me. I didn't know much about the LGBTQ+ spectrum and I believed that to be bisexual I needed to like both genders in *equal* proportion. This confused me greatly, so instead I chose not to name my sexuality.

Of course, now I understand that that isn't the case and that bisexual women can split the percentages wherever they fancy and still have their identity be valid, but at the time it felt like a complete labelling shitshow.

When I started dating my first girlfriend, labels were quickly placed on the table. I thought that being with a woman meant I *had* to identify as a lesbian. It was the closest fit to how I felt and it had been years since I was intimate with a man, so I chose to roll with that and even lean into the label as an identity online with the content I was creating for myself.

Knowing what I know now, though, I've realised that feelings and experiences don't have to be tied to a specific label. What we shared was simply a romantic connection between two women, regardless of what word you use to describe it.

When that relationship ended my attitude to labels shifted again. My mind began to expand to the possibility of 'more'. It felt like I was able to redefine who I was in the way that *I* saw fit, and the opportunity of that felt exciting, yet at the same time a little terrifying, like a 'second' coming out.

Labels were once again on the table, and like a witchy tarot reader I hovered my hands above the options, unsure of what card to pick.

Luckily, since that relationship ended, I've had plenty of time to reflect and become more at ease with fluidity and the idea that who we are and what we want can change over time. But even with that knowledge I still circled around the same questions about who I was and if I even wanted to use a label at all.

My view now, at the time of writing this book, is that I don't particularly resonate with a label – but if I had to pick one, it would be 'fluid'. I am simply 'open' to seeing what naturally unfolds and what life brings my way.

For a long time I thought opening myself up to *more* made me *less* but actually it's quite the opposite. I've always been an extremely open-minded person when it comes to thought processes and ways of thinking. Every interaction, conversation, book I read, podcast I listen to and sexual experience or person I connect with has had a lasting impact on me, and changed the way I show up, act and go forwards, but for a long time I tried to separate how I view life from how I view my sexuality.

I've since realised that to experience true happiness, you need to be aligned with who you are and what you want in *every* aspect of your life. It's a 360-degree approach – no work-arounds or cut-throughs, just pure authenticity, regardless of whether you pick a label or not.

QUEER VOICES

'Labels are important but they aren't rigid. We're allowed to explore, change and grow through our life experiences. The labels I used for myself have changed and that's OK! I love describing myself as queer but if a more accurate label came along, I wouldn't hesitate to change how I label myself.'

'I don't really think people can be labelled as such: there are no two of us who are exactly the same.'

'Labels are helpful but can be misleading and restrictive. I like "queer" best because of the ambiguity. But I also identify with "lesbian", "gay" and "sapphic" when it comes to sexuality. Gender is a whole other matter!'

'I like the term queer. My sexuality is fluid and ever changing. Queer feels like an umbrella term that I can always identify.'

'I can understand that labels are a way to fit in and feel comfortable around people similar to yourself but I have never fitted in. I express myself in many forms. I am just me.'

> **I express myself in many forms. I am just me.**

'If anything, I feel that labels are designed to serve other people's tick-boxing more than they are there to support me . . . but, each to their own: if labels help, good for you! If they don't, I'm here for that, too.'

'I do tend to use lesbian. It very much tells the outside world who I am and instantly lets them know that this woman I am with is not my sister/cousin/friend. The trans label I use less. As a cis-passing trans woman the world is a scary place and I tend to hide that, even from people who I consider as friends. It makes me sad that I cannot be proud of that label for personal safety reasons.'

Don't be swayed by stereotypes

People love to categorise and label things. It's in our nature. Early humans used categorisation and labelling to identify safe and dangerous things, which was crucial for survival. Today (depending on where you live, of course) fewer of us are on the lookout daily for dangerous predators, but this way of 'being' is still embedded in how we use language, communicate with each other and encourage the use of labels as a way to organise and co-ordinate our behaviour.

With this categorisation comes 'grouping', where people are placed into systems based on common features, behaviours and traits (i.e. stereotypes).

Lesbians come with their own set of stereotypes, as do bisexuals, gay men and many more 'sub-groups' of the queer community, but that *doesn't* mean that you need to accept or adhere to those if you choose to identify that way.

> While there's real joy in coming together and being part of a group (and we should absolutely allow ourselves that), it doesn't change the fact that we're all our own people and allowed to express ourselves how we wish to.

Are labels helpful or hurtful?

Choosing whether or not to use a label to describe your sexuality can feel like a huge decision, and it's not always an easy one. There are potential benefits and challenges of both identifying with a label and electing not to. But hopefully by weighing the pros and cons, you can reflect on what feels most authentic and supportive for you in your journey. Remember, there's no right or wrong here, only what works best for your unique experience.

Here are some things to consider:

Pros of choosing a label:

- **Clarity and self-understanding** – Labels can help you articulate your feelings and attractions, giving language to what might otherwise feel confusing or undefined.
- **Community and belonging** – Identifying with a label often connects you to communities of people with similar experiences, providing support and solidarity.
- **Validation** – Putting a name to your identity can be affirming, reducing internal conflict and increasing self-acceptance.
- **Communication** – Labels make it easier to explain your identity to others, which can improve relationships and create understanding.
- **Empowerment** – For many, claiming a label is an act of pride and resistance against societal norms.

Cons of choosing a label:

- **Feeling boxed in** – Labels can sometimes feel restrictive, making you worry that you need to fit perfectly into a predefined category.

LABELS

- **Changing identities** – Your feelings and identity may evolve, leading to confusion or anxiety if a chosen label no longer fits.
- **Judgement and stigma** – Labels can expose you to discrimination or misunderstanding from others who don't accept or respect your identity.
- **Overwhelm from options** – The growing number of labels can feel confusing or overwhelming, making it hard to pick one that 'fits'.

Pros of not using a label:

- **Freedom and flexibility** – Avoiding labels can let you explore your identity without pressure to conform or explain yourself.
- **Less external pressure** – Without a label, you may feel less burdened by others' expectations or judgements.
- **Personal focus** – You can focus on your feelings and experiences without the need to categorise them for others.
- **Rejecting binaries** – Not labelling can be a way to resist rigid societal structures around sexuality.

Cons of not using a label:

- **Lack of language** – Without a label, it can be harder to communicate your identity to others, which might lead to misunderstandings.
- **Isolation** – You might miss out on community or support networks often organised around shared labels, though not using one doesn't mean you shouldn't be included.
- **Internal confusion** – Not having a label might sometimes feel like you're avoiding your identity or stuck in uncertainty.
- **External pressure** – Society often expects people to 'pick a side', which can lead to frustration or questioning from friends, family or partners.

Labels can be powerful tools for self-expression, finding community and gaining personal clarity, but they're not essential for everyone. Whether you embrace a specific label, move fluidly between a few or decide not to use any at all, the most important thing is that your choice feels authentic and reflects who you are as you grow and evolve.

It's OK to change your mind

If you've already chosen a label to describe your sexuality but lately feel like it no longer fits, then you're definitely not alone. Changing how you identify can stir up a lot of emotions – confusion, doubt, even guilt – as if you're undoing something you once firmly believed. It can feel like stepping back or starting over, and that's a tough place to be.

But what if changing your label isn't a setback at all, but a natural part of understanding yourself more deeply?

For me, the air definitely lifted around labelling my sexuality as soon as I started to talk about my feelings, but I still felt scared to admit that what I'd wanted had changed. It had felt for a while like a failing on my part – that I thought I knew who I was, yet somehow had been wrong. It temporarily shook my confidence and belief system and made me feel lost.

Changing your label, or questioning it, can bring up fears of being misunderstood, judged or even rejected. When you've spent a long time moving through the world in a particular way, and when your friends or family have come to see that version of you as 'normal', any shift in that identity can feel disruptive.

When I started exploring my sexuality again in my early 30s, after having relationships with women, I felt some strange emotions bubbling up. One of the biggest was the fear that my identity might suddenly become 'less valid' and that others would see me as *confused* if I allowed myself to explore the idea of fluidity.

Fluidity, by the way, is the description I've landed on (a label that isn't really a label at all). It simply means I'm open-minded. I'm a queer woman, attracted to women, but if life or my brain ever threw me a curveball, I wouldn't immediately reject it.

In my opinion fluidity doesn't make anyone's identity less real or attraction less valid. In fact, if anything, it shows emotional intelligence, confidence and honesty (mic drop).

But reaching that point wasn't linear. I went through the whole mental obstacle course: worrying that calling myself bisexual might make me sound 'greedy'; then worrying I wasn't 'gay enough' to use the word lesbian; and then, while writing this chapter and unpacking new feelings, temporarily fearing that being open to 'more' might somehow make me 'less' in the LGBTQ+ space.

Eventually, though, I realised that even if people have opinions about your identity, those opinions don't have to carry any weight.

And as the months passed, and I kept having conversations with more and more people, both inside and outside the LGBTQ+ community, I had a genuinely life-changing realisation:

It's just not that deep

You're allowed to change your mind and explore different ways of identifying as many times as you need to. And if something doesn't feel right along the way, you're allowed to shift, adjust, or completely reinvent.

There should be zero shame in self-exploration when it comes to identity.

And once we accept that doubts are part of the journey, it becomes much easier to quiet them and move forwards with confidence in who we are. There will always be moments when we question if we're 'enough', and that goes far beyond identity or labels. But the more rooted we are in *who* we are, the less power those doubts have to shake us or steer our path.

Knowing yourself and what you want is *hot* – and keeping up the dialogue around it is, in my opinion, even *hotter*.

To that end, here are some final thoughts on labels from my queer community:

QUEER VOICES

'I went from bi to gay. I very quickly realised (within a month of the sapphic epiphany) that I didn't actually like men at all, but needed a second to come to terms with it.'

'I haven't changed my label since coming out almost 10 years ago. However, I've felt pressure to do so: to go from identifying as bi to calling myself a lesbian. Biphobia and bi erasure are sadly alive and well in the community of queer women and we have to fight that.'

'For me, "bisexual" was a stepping stone, but that doesn't mean bisexuality isn't valid; it absolutely is. My journey just happened to land in a different place.'

'I'm slightly more open to a more fluid sexuality now we have, in this country at least [the UK], experienced some progressive political change. Back in the 1980s and 90s a lot of the equality rhetoric was framed around binary identities. It was sort of useful for explaining things in the sort of rigid terms the law works with, despite being rather reductive about something as expansive as human sexuality.'

'I think I've arrived back at queer now, because to me, queer isn't just a sexuality, it's political. Being queer is about rejecting societal norms, and championing those who don't fit into the cisheteropatriarchy too.'

Some people find a label that fits and stick with it for life, and if that's you, that's completely valid. But for others, trying to land on a single word might feel limiting, like forcing yourself into a box that was never quite made for you.

The truth is that connection, attraction and identity don't always follow a fixed pattern. They can be fluid, shifting over time, and that's OK.

As you move through life, what feels right might change. And sometimes, what feels right might even surprise you.

Reassessing your identity isn't something to fear or feel ashamed of: it's a sign of self-awareness. A sign that you're evolving.

Remember, labels are tools, not rules. They're meant to support your understanding of yourself, not restrict it. They can offer community and clarity, but they're not requirements.

Whether you find one label that feels like home, shift between several or decide not to use any at all, your journey is yours. It's valid. It's real. And it doesn't need to look like anyone else's.

So trust yourself. Let your identity unfold in its own time. Keep choosing what feels true, whatever that looks like for you.

THREE

Connections

Connection is at the heart of so much in life, and it's especially important when you're navigating your identity as a queer woman. Whether you're just starting to understand yourself or have been exploring for a while, building meaningful connections is vital – and it starts with the one you build with yourself.

For this reason, I want to begin this chapter by exploring what it means to connect first with yourself: why that internal relationship is so important for feeling grounded and confident, and how self-acceptance lays the foundation for everything that follows. Coming out doesn't automatically make you feel whole or certain, ready to be seen by the world. For many of us, it's just the beginning – and self-connection is the first step.

It can feel incredibly challenging and daunting, especially when you're newly out. Not knowing where to find others like you – people who *actually* understand what you're going through – can make the whole process feel isolating. But we're not going to let that happen. Because once you've learned to truly connect with yourself, reaching out to others will feel lighter, easier, and ultimately set you on a path toward a deeper sense of belonging.

That's why the second part of this chapter is all about finding your people within the community in a *platonic* way. I'll dive into my top tips (and all the juicy things to consider) about romantic connections later in the book. For now, think of this chapter as your starting point, a space to explore what it means to belong, from the inside out.

The topics we're going to explore are:

- The process of connecting with yourself, including practical (no bullshit) suggestions for how to actually do this, such as self-development, therapy, listening to podcasts/reading books, taking the time to reflect, and more
- Why it's important to connect with others in the community, and how to *actually* find and be a part of this space.

MY STORY

After coming out at 21, I was relieved and excited to start a new chapter, but at the same time, I moved through life feeling like a 14-year-old who had just hit puberty again, with my thoughts running at 3000 miles per hour, like a chaotic movie in my mind: *Who the f*ck am I? How do I want to dress? Who do I want to have sex with? How do you even have sex with another woman? Do I even like my hair? Do I want to get a tattoo? What kind of person do I think is hot, and who am I just pre-conditioned by society to think is hot? And more importantly, how the f*ck do I figure all of this out?*

In a nutshell, I was *spiralling*.

One of the hardest things for me to grasp during that period of exploration, which only added to my confusion, was how society portrayed queer women. Back in 2015, when I came out, representation on the internet, TV and film was significantly limited, and social platforms like TikTok and Instagram were just getting started. There were few visuals or narratives about what lesbian, bisexual and queer women looked like, and I often felt like I hadn't received the memo or didn't quite fit the 'brief'.

It seemed like there were only a handful of ways to present yourself as a queer woman, and none of them truly resonated with me, which, like someone scrolling LinkedIn job ads, made me question if I was even right for the role...

For me there was a fear that I was too 'feminine' to be allowed to be into other women and I was frightened that all of this impending 'exploration' might mean that I had to give up parts of me that I really liked (my skincare routine, wardrobe and jewellery, to name a few). Looking back, it feels ridiculous to even think that the process of exploring your identity would mean that you need to ditch who you are, but at the time the fear around dutifully releasing parts of me that I didn't want to give up, in the name of becoming 'gay', was *very* real.

The fear was strong because not only did the way I outwardly present make me feel safe, happy and confident but it made me, *me*.

You might be experiencing similar thoughts (potentially not about the loss of skincare, but in your own way) and that's completely valid. Perhaps you don't want to give up the clothes that make you feel like *you*, whether that's your impeccable boot collection, or your obsession with oversized jumpers. Or perhaps it's less about the external and more around how you internally feel about wanting to maintain parts of a past identity (like the friendship groups you've built, the routines that keep you grounded, or the hobbies that have shaped your sense of self as you step into a new queer identity). All of these thoughts and fears are valid.

No matter what choices you make about your identity or expression, I believe that the core parts of who you are should always stay with you. Otherwise, you risk trading your authenticity for something that doesn't truly fit, and compromising who you are will never serve you in the long run.

Another part of exploring my sexuality that I seriously grappled with was whether I was stepping into an 'improved' and more 'confident' version of myself or taking up behaviours and making changes to my appearance because I thought that's what I *needed* to do to prove to myself and others that I was indeed worthy of being part of the LGBTQ+ community.

In short, I had no real frame of reference for who this new version of me was: what felt genuine and true versus what felt forced or performative. That lack of clarity left me feeling constantly on edge, defensive and worried about what people would think of me.

During summer 2015, after I had moved to London full time, I was at a rather dull networking evening that my boss had sent me to in a bid to appease our clients and show face. Luckily, there was a well-stocked buffet table at the back of the room that I and a large group of male attendees instinctively gravitated towards.

Usually, being surrounded mostly by men at such an event might put a woman off, but not me. Perhaps this was because A) I felt safe from judgement (as in my massively generalised opinion men seemed less perceptive as a gender to the emotional struggles I was going through at the time, and it was easier to hide how I felt); B) there was a part of me that felt like I needed the validation of male attention; and C) simply that they happened to also be the people who felt awkward at social events too, and the buffet table was our shared safe space.

Whatever the cause, on this particular night I stood ramming crisps into my mouth and drinking a beer from the bottle. I had chosen to wear a skirt in a bid not to look like what I thought was a 'raging homosexual' (even though I have since scrapped every skirt I own and never put one on my legs again; there's nothing wrong with skirts – they're just not for me) yet even in an attempt to disguise myself, I felt incredibly sensitive.

'It's refreshing to see a woman drink a beer from the bottle,' one guy said, while jabbing another and laughing.

I looked down at my hands and immediately felt like the choices I'd made for consuming my drink were a massive giveaway of my sexuality. *Women don't drink beer from a bottle*, I thought. *Women aren't like this – women are supposed to be dainty and I'm masculine*. I could feel my heart starting to race as the thoughts swirled around my head.

'I couldn't find a glass,' I snapped back.

They all looked a little perplexed.

It was a wildly inappropriate comment to make to me in the first place, but their words had hit a particular kind of nerve.

Drinking beer from the bottle seemed like a manly/lesbian/gay thing to do, yet it was also totally *me*, but because I wasn't sure who 'me' actually was any more, I perceived their comments as a judgement. I proceeded to run off, lock myself in the toilet, sob into some damp tissue (smattered with flakes of pastry from a sausage roll I'd consumed just moments earlier) and eventually leave out of the back exit in shame.

This behaviour, categorised by my sense of shame, but also intrigue for who I might be, carried on for a number of months as I navigated my way through the chaotic journey of getting to know myself. My inner monologue went into overdrive. It was shouting at me, questioning everything: *Do I actually want to f*ck a woman?* Could I have a relationship with a woman? Or was this just about hanging out with the guys, cracking open some beers, and bonding over how much we love women ... then maybe end up f*cking one of them instead?*
[cue further spiralling]

---

1) Connecting with yourself

This chaotic stage of finding yourself after you come out can feel absolutely wild and if you're in it right now, you might be asking yourself what you can do to start the process of unpacking your feelings in a systematic and level-headed way before you internally combust.

So let's just tap the brake for a second before we go any further.

It's not a case of marching around with a rainbow flag or grinding up on someone to the soundtrack of Lady Gaga to find an answer (although those things will probably help) but starting with little steps to calm your nervous system, gain clarity and move forwards. The tools below are intended to help you connect more deeply to yourself and begin to understand the emotions and feelings that might be coming up for you during this period.

Therapy

My first suggestion is therapy. Having someone listen to you in a non-biased, judgement-free way is incredibly useful to help you understand your emotions, particularly when it comes to sexuality and identity.

Just like a broken arm or a migraine that won't go away, it's important that you check out any mental health issues with a professional. They can hold space for you and advise you in ways that your family, friends and co-workers can't. Yes, you need to find a good one and yes, sometimes that means spending money, but there are also plenty of free schemes through organisations, work and charities that you can explore, too.

Finding a therapist who identifies as LGBTQ+ can also be a game changer. They will likely understand you on a deeper level, meaning that you can connect quicker and immediately enter a space that feels safe and secure.

Whoever you choose, you need to build a solid relationship with them, as this might be one of your first experiences of vulnerability outside your trusted circle and that should be an honour for someone to listen to and hold.

Write an 'Enjoy' list

When I was struggling with accepting my sexuality after I'd come out, I had periods when I felt extremely low. I found it hard to find joy in the mundane and I often felt like time blurred as I noticed myself eating the same thing, walking the same route to and from work and thinking the same debilitating thoughts.

The cycle of trudging through your days needs to be broken (seriously!) and rewired with positive experiences, places, people and things.

Breaking out of a negative or monotonous mental cycle is crucial because our brains are wired to form habits, both good and bad, through repeated patterns of thought and behaviour. When you deliberately introduce positive experiences or reminders of joy, even briefly, you start to create new neural pathways. This process, called neuroplasticity, allows your brain to rewire itself over time, making positive thought patterns more accessible and automatic.

This is something I like to challenge myself to do regularly, and I call it my 'Enjoy' list. It's as simple as pulling up the notes app on your phone or going old school with pen and paper and thinking about the things that make you feel happy.

I understand this might be hard to do if you're feeling extremely low, but even finding the smallest of things that you can identify and turn to when you feel down will make a world of difference. They don't have to light your soul on fire, but instead bring you a sense of calm, safety and security.

It will likely start small and get bigger as time progresses. Here are my lists, to illustrate how much the world opens up when you allow yourself to experience more.

My 'Enjoy' list at 21:

- Listening to music
- Watching TV
- Reading psychology articles and books
- Taking photos

My 'Enjoy' list in my 30s:

- Hosting dinner parties
- Reading psychology books
- Dancing
- Red wine
- Kissing
- House music
- Karaoke
- Hot sauce
- Looking out of a plane window
- Hiking
- Swimming in the ocean
- The smell of roses
- The sound of other people's laughter

Tap into podcasts, books and social media

If you're feeling unsettled and searching for answers about how you might be feeling, the internet can be a powerful tool, allowing you to learn from others and open your mind to experiences beyond the bubble you currently sit in. Exploring different stories and perspectives can help you unpack parts of yourself, challenging old beliefs, sparking new insights and encouraging growth in understanding your own sexual identity.

This is a topic I could easily bang on about for days, but to keep it brief: please use social media intentionally and mindfully. Seek out and follow accounts of authentic people whose content uplifts you and makes you feel good about yourself. Surrounding yourself with positive, relatable voices can nurture your journey towards self-acceptance and clarity.

Also, be cautious not to drown yourself in endless scrolling through curated highlight reels that only serve to make you feel inadequate or confused. Remember, what you see online is often a polished version of reality, not the full picture. Using social media with purpose can help you feel more connected to yourself and the community, rather than isolated or overwhelmed.

We are lucky to have access to many LGBTQ+ creators who are making waves with their content, so tap into that and use your energy to listen to what they have to say. Their life stories and vulnerability will help you to feel more seen and hopefully offer up potential solutions to your worries.

Reflexercise

One of my favourite activities to do when I want to understand the thoughts I'm having on a deeper emotional level is putting my phone on airplane mode and going for a long walk to do some reflexercise (reflecting and exercise combined).

I clear my schedule to march around in silence for long periods of time so I can listen to what's truly going on deep down that needs to surface. I also mutter the thoughts out loud as I stomp around, arguing and posing questions to my inner monologue, until I reach a conclusion about what I want to do next.

This activity does more than just make you look like a crazy person and release any built-up tension – it also *literally* allows your brain the chance to process information.

When we walk, our eyes make lateral movements, constantly sending signals to our brain, updating it about where we are and what dangers might be in our peripheral vision. Lateral eye movements are also linked to our cognition, memory and emotional processing. Research indicates that these movements can influence memory vividness and emotionality. A meta-analysis by Houben *et al.* interestingly found that performing eye movements during memory retrieval can decrease the vividness of negative autobiographical memories, suggesting a role in emotional processing.

To put it simply, if you want to understand how you feel about something that has happened in the past, work through potential solutions to those feelings and feel better about it all, then it's better to be on the move than sitting down.

And the great thing about it is that it doesn't matter how far you walk – lateral eye movements kick in immediately. I personally prefer to allow myself at least an hour of moving my body (perhaps an indication of how much I have going on inside my head), but you might only need 20 minutes.

Spending time alone is key. So many of us are scared to spend time alone for fear of what might 'come up' when we take away the distractions, but I firmly believe that sitting (or walking) in that silence, albeit challenging if we're struggling with our identity, is one of the most transformative things we can do.

You simply *cannot* make big life shifts and decisions if you have too much noise going on around you.

Want to be convinced immediately? Look up from this book right now and stare at something. I'd now like you to picture a purple horse.

Struggling to do that? Now try closing your eyes.

I would bet my life savings on you being able to process and develop what a purple horse looks like once you shut out the external distractions and turn your focus inwards.

We need to create a clearing in our external *and* internal environment so that our thoughts can catch up with us. We need to look at them, explore them and ask them the hard questions. Then when the answers eventually come, listen, accept and take action on the truth we discover, no matter how hard that might be.

I asked my community of queer women about the ways that they connected to their identity and began to unravel their sexuality after they came out. The answers were very interesting!

QUEER VOICES

'As a bisexual who came out while being in a monogamous relationship with a man, I didn't choose to explore my sexuality with having actual sexual experiences with women. Instead, I cultivated my queer identity by listening to queer music, watching TV shows and movies with LGBTQ+ creators and reading books by gay authors.'

'I watched anything and everything that had even a vague lesbian storyline! I desperately craved representation tucked away in a rural Welsh community where I was definitely the only gay in the village!'

'I went on Tinder and dated as many women as I could have time for!'

'Once I came out, I sought queer spaces: small Prides, LGBTQ+ events and online communities. Slowly I built a life where being a lesbian wasn't shameful, but joyful.'

> **Slowly I built a life where being a lesbian wasn't shameful, but joyful.**

'My fashion sense was one of the first big ways I wanted to express my sexuality when I came out. I bought all the sneaker loafers and asked all my friends if I looked "gay". I'm also so obsessed with lesbian musical artists. I love hearing a song by a woman about a woman, and I don't have to change it in my head from the heteronormative songs we grew up with.'

'My biggest relief and sense of "this is me" was when I was 18. My mum wouldn't let me cut my hair and it was very long. She agreed I could have it cut off when I was 18 so I cut it VERY short. I turned up at prom and I wore a pinstripe suit, hair gone. No one recognised me. It was the start of a journey, feeling comfortable in my skin. Over the years this fades, you redesign and keep going. But that day, that feeling. WOW.'

2) Connecting with others

The next thing we can do to help connect more deeply with ourselves is actually a surprising one: connect with *others*.

Humans are wired for connection because, from an evolutionary standpoint, a lone human had significantly less chance of surviving than one who was part of a group or tribe. Early humans relied on pooling resources, co-operative hunting and collective protection to increase their survival odds. These behaviours were essential to human survival and success, as they enabled shared resources, protection from threats and improved care for offspring.

Although we no longer depend on friends to keep the fire going or hunt for food (although sometimes I send my mates to the corner shop if I'm hungover), the underlying principle remains the same: we are stronger, safer and feel more supported when we are together.

In addition, beyond evolutionary survival advantages, humans, especially women, respond to stress by seeking social support and nurturing relationships, a process described by psychologist Shelley Taylor as the 'tend and befriend' response.

Unlike the traditional fight-or-flight reaction, this biological and psychological mechanism encourages connection and caregiving behaviours that promote group cohesion and safety. This theory highlights how deeply ingrained our need for social bonds is (particularly for women), demonstrating that belongingness is not just beneficial but a fundamental response to stress and threat.

So why is this important for the LGBTQ+ community then?

Forming connections is good for us in many ways. It:

1. **Helps form a secure base to launch from** – You can try new things and know that you can retreat to people who understand and support you, providing a safety net so that risk-taking (aka growth) feels less scary.
2. **Provides back-up against self-doubt** – When you're cut off from the world, you can sometimes start to judge yourself as 'different', 'bad' or 'not worthwhile'. Having a community around you means that those negative stories lose power and belonging rewrites the inner script to 'I'm valued here'.
3. **Boosts mood** – Loneliness drags mood down, leaving you less energised, flatter and more irritable. Being around supportive people lifts mood, resources and energy and gives you the confidence to speak up and shine.
4. **Builds resilience** – Connection is the antidote to fear. With a group behind you, you're much more willing to put yourself out

there and take risks. That lived confidence snowballs and with each small win, your brain is convinced and thinks, *Hey, I can do this!*
5. **Is good for your physical health** – Isolation triggers stress responses (sleep issues, appetite swings, weaker immunity). Reconnection calms the system so your body isn't screaming 'danger' when you step into the world, but rather approaching it from a less-heightened and calmer state.

Personally, as soon as I started to connect with others (queer and non-queer) my brain started to rewire and shift from a mindset that I was someone no one cared about, to being someone who was seen and celebrated, and a part of me began to heal.

When we think about making new connections in the queer community, our minds often jump straight to dating. And while meeting someone in this capacity can be a really fun part of being a queer woman, it's not the *only* thing that can bring you joy and confidence.

In my personal experience, the very first and most crucial step to happiness is building a solid, supportive platonic community around you. As an LGBTQ+ person, having a group of good people you can rely on – friends who understand you, uplift you and celebrate you – is what truly empowers you to take on the world with confidence.

My guide to finding queer friends

When I was growing up I always imagined making friends (much like a '90s movie, where you have multitrack phone calls and all wear matching outfits) as a one-stop shop. I thought I needed to find a group of people that I bonded with, join the clique and then I'd be set for life.

But, funnily enough that's not how it works.

For most of us, especially living in the world we do now, it's a rarity to find a large group of people that you can hang out with on a regular basis, yet we still cling to this as an ideal of friendship and connection. The modern-day reality is that unless you have access to the usual places where you would find groups of communities such as school, university, an office, sports teams or community groups, we are more likely to encounter people that we vibe with on a 1–1 basis. It's also true that even if we do have access to large groups of people, we might not actually want to hang out with them or they might not want to hang out with us (it happens, you're not always going to be people's cup of tea), so, for most of us, individual 'curation' of a group of people is how we structure the connections in our lives.

When we talk about making friends in the Queer space we often hear the phrase 'The community will welcome you with open arms', and although generally speaking we are a very welcoming bunch, much like making friends as an adult, it still takes *effort*. It's very unlikely (although not impossible) that you'll wander into a bar and find a group of 10 Queer women you like and that's you set for life (mainly because you'll probably end up sleeping with at least 3 of them, and their ex partners, and you'll want to quite quickly expand your circle).

The sexuality thing always seems to surprise people when I talk about my friendship group too. Weirdly, people expect me to have a gigantic group of queer influencer friends that I bounce around with like some kind of K-pop group, shunning the straights and pushing the gay agenda. As fun as this sounds to do for a few hours, let me assure you that's not the case.

My friendship group consists of people from all walks of life, sexualities, genders, backgrounds, ages and more.

It does not matter *how* the people you spend time with identify, what matters is that you find **true** connection where acceptance and love is reciprocated. That being said it's definitely important to have queer friends added into your mix (whether you are newly out or have been out for some time), as the conversations that you have are going to be beneficial to your growth.

It's incredibly important to find a space to communicate with others who have experienced what you're feeling and in turn allow yourself the opportunity to feel seen and held in a different way than you might experience with your friends who are allies.

So, how do you go about making these meaningful connections and finding your tribe? Let me share some guidance below to help you navigate this journey:

Events and groups

If you're looking to make queer friends, a great place to start is by following your interests and attending events or meet-up groups that genuinely appeal to you. Not only will you meet people who share similar passions, but you'll also be stepping out of your comfort zone, into new spaces, new experiences and, ultimately, a more open-minded headspace.

There are so many different types of events and groups out there for queer women, and thankfully, the range is growing. We're moving past the idea that the only options are either 3a.m. nightclub chaos or whispering over prose poetry (though both are totally valid!). There's a whole spectrum in between, and somewhere in there, you'll likely find your people.

You might discover book events, speed 'friend' dating, football teams, wine nights, creative workshops, walking groups . . . the list goes on. Each time you show up to something new, you're not just building social connections, you're strengthening your sense of self and growing your confidence.

If you don't live in a city or large town, it can feel tougher when events are fewer and farther between. But connection is still possible – you just have to meet your local community where they are. Maybe hiking isn't your thing, but if there's a walking group nearby, try going along once. You never know who you'll meet or what unexpected connection might spark.

Also, don't be afraid to travel. Even if it's just once every couple of months, heading to events in nearby towns or cities can widen your circle and give you fresh opportunities to connect outside of your usual environment.

The most important thing? Start small, stay curious and keep showing up. The right people will find you, and you'll find more of *yourself* in the process too. So that's my advice, but let's find out what other queer women have to say:

QUEER VOICES

'I've found the best way is to put yourself out there, and see what queer events are going on in your city. It can be scary at first, especially if you're by yourself, but once you go to one event and talk to one or two people it just follows from there! Many people tend to go to multiple events so it's really nice to see the same people again and build up friendships from there.'

CONNECTIONS

Go to places that centre queer joy

'Go to places that centre queer joy: festivals, arts, nature groups, community nights. Being queer is one part of you, so find things that you're actually interested in. You don't need to go to bars or club nights if that isn't for you. You'll also make more lasting friendships with people you meet in places of shared interest.'

'I always encourage people to attend queer events alone. It can be frightening but attending a show where you can simply watch and not feel pressure to mingle can be freeing.'

'I've found it a little difficult being a bit older and having a small close friend/family group to go out to queer spaces. I'm not a big clubber and a lot of my friends are married with kids so they have busy lives anyway. I did join a meet-up group and go to a few events but never found anything I stuck with. So I'm still working on this.'

The internet

Social media is a fantastic way to connect with other people. It opens up an entire world at your fingertips and allows you to have conversations with other people without the need to be physically in the same space. For queer women, this can be particularly useful as you start to find a community and connect with others.

Instagram is great for finding out about local events and meet-ups happening near you. Yes, you have to go digging for these accounts but usually the algorithm will lend a helping hand with that and point you in the right direction. Look out for LGBTQ+ creators who host regular meet-ups, picnics or parties (there are many of them). Give them a follow and make sure that you're aware of when these meet-ups are happening so you can plan to attend.

WhatsApp groups and group chats are also common ways for queer women to hear about what is happening in the community and to keep in touch with each other. Admittedly these are a little harder to infiltrate as a newly out queer, but usually invites come as you get to know people – so make sure you're getting yourself out there and talking to others!

At the time of writing this chapter I've just returned from a picnic in central London – an afternoon in Hyde Park that brought together the queer community for quite literally what it says on the tin . . . a picnic. There were blankets and loaves of bread and cheese boards everywhere. It was wholesome and gorgeous.

As my picnic example demonstrates, people are now using platforms like TikTok, Instagram and many other social spaces to bring people together *offline*. People are hungry for real-life connection and this, in my opinion, is where social media is a force for good: reaching the masses and turning that connection into something that can last and is tangible in the real world.

Of course, social media is also a place where you can form one-on-one connections with others and friendships can also blossom. But don't just take my word for it – here's what others have to say about friendship:

QUEER VOICES

Everyone is going through something. Always approach the ones hiding in the corner!

'I've made many friends online, I recommend putting out positivity in the comments and follow people you want to be friends with! But don't be pushy!'

'Message boards and social media helped me find community when I didn't have it locally. It was a lifeline as a teenager, but I did do some silly and unsafe things because we just didn't know what we now know about online safety. Stay mindful that people present an image of themselves online; social media isn't real life.'

'Be brave, don't judge and be you. Everyone is going through something. Always approach the ones hiding in the corner! Do it.'

'I mean I wouldn't be talking to you now if we hadn't connected online! I think slipping into DMs is such a brave thing but also be mindful that it can open you up to unnecessary attention. It's a hard balance: trust your gut, find communities, LGBTQ+ spokespeople and just be kind. If you wouldn't say it face to face then don't type it is my advice!'

Organised travel groups

Group travel is a great way to throw yourself directly into an environment where everyone is open to forming new connections, and the pressure of wondering if you'll look out of place for striking up a conversation with someone new is entirely off.

In 2024 a good friend of mine who is also a creator and I decided to team up and create a 'gaycation' to Costa Rica for our online communities. Open to only queer women, nonbinary and trans travellers, we put out posts inviting people to join us on a crazy adventure across rainforests, volcanoes and black-sand beaches, and to our surprise 10 people signed up for the trip. We met on a rainy evening in San José and bundled ourselves into a minibus, cracked a few jokes and instantly became best friends.

Since then I have continued to run trips for queer travellers. In collaboration with a travel company who organises all of the details, I host vacations to LGBTQ+-friendly destinations all around the world and invite my community to join me.

Group travel is more than just yapping, laughing and playing silly music, though – these trips truly heal parts of ourselves that sometimes we don't even know needed healing in the first place.

Every time I return from running a gaycation I'm on a total high. Seeing queer women make connections with each other, sharing their vulnerability and truly growing, gives me more joy that I can explain.

It's entirely the essence of what 'community' stands for: creating a space where nobody in the world can f*ck with us, where we're unstoppable, full of joy and changed for the better.

Ironically, it has nothing to do with *where* we are in the world and everything to do with *who* we are with instead (although of course I make sure to pick places that are fun too!).

Travel is an incredible tool for getting to know yourself and others and it doesn't always have to be done by leaving your country. There are plenty of queer-led day trips and tours, hiking groups and more, which with a little bit of research you might be able to join and start exploring yourself.

To find out how travel can be beneficial, I asked my community of queer women for their views:

QUEER VOICES

'I loved not having to explain myself as a nonbinary person. I knew I would be welcome in a queer travel group, and that led me to open up more quickly.'

'The friends I met as part of a queer group travelling were so important for me. As that child who never fitted in, into that young adult who never fitted in, to suddenly feel at home among a group of women who I came to love was so validating. Travel is intense but a rewarding shared experience. Seeing a new waterfall or beautiful vista links you to others in a way that a mere club cannot.'

'Everyone has a similar story to tell, about how they felt being in the closet and how their journey came about. In many other travel groups I've been with there isn't much interaction and you just get transported around to locations of interest, [but] travelling in queer groups is different.'

'Travelling with a group of queer individuals enabled everyone to connect on a much deeper level. We spent the week laughing, crying, being vulnerable yet safe, sharing personal experiences, asking for advice . . . all while being authentically ourselves. The destination may have been foreign but the group felt like home.'

Pride events

Going to your first queer event when you're freshly out or even questioning can be an incredibly daunting experience, but it can also be completely euphoric.

In 2018, three years after I came out, I went to my first Pride event. I felt sick before I left the house because it was the first time that I was outwardly saying, 'Here I am and I'm not straight!', which wasn't something I'd ever been comfortable putting so outwardly on display.

My outfit consisted of a red crop top, hot pants and white Converse high tops. The only rainbow I wore was a small band on my socks, but it felt like enough of a step to signal I was part of the community. As I walked through town I noticed people were staring at me and I started to crumble. I wondered if I was experiencing my first homophobic incident after only walking two paces down the road, until I clocked myself in a shop window and saw that my hot pants were riding so high that you could see my arse cheeks, and realised that perhaps *that* was the reason I was getting so much attention.

It's totally fine and normal not to want to wrap yourself in a giant Pride flag or dip yourself head to toe in glitter if you're not ready or dislike the attention. You can be gay without looking like a diva, but you can also be a diva if you want to. Again, there's no *right* or *wrong* way to do this.

That said, I really recommend you bring a friend with you to attend Pride. It might be a very emotional experience for you, especially if you've been struggling, and having that support is invaluable. If you don't have anyone to go with you then you can find communities via meet-up apps, Instagram, TikTok or even local LGBTQ+ centres and charities. You're never alone!

Here's how some others in my community experienced their first Pride events:

QUEER VOICES

'The first Pride I ever went to was in Galway in the west of Ireland. There were maybe 100 people at it; we had such a laugh. I'll never forget the amount of love that brought to my world that day, in technicolour.'

'I used to attend Pride alone. I would go watch the parade and just feel so envious of everyone being their authentic selves freely and proudly. After coming out I realised why I had always enjoyed attending alone: I found my family.'

'I went to Cardiff Pride and I had no idea what to expect but it was a really fun day! It was before marriage equality, and I remember seeing a huge queue at the blessing tent, where queer couples could have their relationship witnessed before the law actually caught up! The mix of celebration and the quiet defiance that runs through the LGBTQ+ community made my first Pride really memorable.'

'1992. I marched with my girlfriend and attended a free party in Brockwell Park. Kissing and holding hands in public felt very radical. That part of London still means a lot to me.'

'It was by accident. I was still married, not really connected to the community in any way. By pure chance I had booked a matinee theatre ticket in London on the same day as Pride. I came out of the performance and practically walked in the parade. So I just stood and watched it on my own for a while, and it was lovely to see even though I felt quite disconnected from it in some ways.'

'I was 18, living in Chicago for college, and went with the university's LGBTQ+ group. I hadn't been to many parades in general, having grown up in a small town in rural Tennessee. Going to a Pride parade in Chicago seemed so surreal. There was so much colour, good vibes, and a sense of belonging.'

One final message about connection

True self-acceptance begins with turning inwards. Sometimes, when you pause, suspend your fears and focus on connecting with yourself, you return to those fears to find they've shrunk, or even transformed completely.

Taking time to reflect on who you are helps you build a stronger foundation of self-understanding and self-worth.

But this journey isn't one you have to make alone. In fact, connecting with others can be one of the most powerful ways to deepen your connection with yourself. Being seen, heard and understood by others, especially within the queer community, can reflect parts of you that you may not have fully recognised or embraced yet.

Confidence often grows not in isolation, but in the shared experience of community.

So don't pass up opportunities to start conversations, try something new or step outside your comfort zone. Whether it's friendship, chosen family or broader community spaces, every connection has the potential to support your growth.

Whatever form it takes, connection is always worth your while, because together, we are *always* stronger.

FOUR

Dating

Throw anything my way and I've probably seen it, made out with it, taken an international flight for it... or torn my hair out over it.

Welcome to dating women!

If you're reading this, chances are you're either stepping into this world for the first time or revisiting it with a fresh perspective. Either way, deep breath, you're not alone.

Dating as a queer woman comes with its own unique blend of magic and mystery. For many, especially those who've recently come out or are still exploring their identity, entering this space can feel like being dropped into a game where no one quite handed you the rulebook. You might be wondering...

What actually counts as a date?
Who's meant to make the first move?
Does she actually like me?
Why is everyone talking about U-Hauling?
And how the hell do I flirt?

It's normal to feel anxious. You're navigating new terrain, and it's OK if your heart races a little (or a lot), or if you replay the whole evening 25 times in your head after it ends. Queer dating culture is fun, yes, but it can also be layered, emotionally intense and wildly unpredictable (in both the best and worst ways).

The truth is, we often build dating up in our heads before we even give ourselves the chance to try. We overthink, overanalyse, panic and worry if we're 'doing it right'. But dating isn't a test. It's a space for discovery. Of other people, but more importantly, of yourself. What lights you up, what makes you feel safe, what gives you butterflies and what subtly tells you, *No, this isn't for me.*

So let's make this feel a little less overwhelming.

In this chapter, we'll cover the essentials – not just the logistics of dating, but the emotional side of it, too:

- How dating a woman is different to dating a man
- How to figure out what you're actually looking for
- Where to meet women in non-pressured, authentic ways
- How to flirt
- How to tell if she's into you or just being friendly
- The practicalities of going on a date (and lock in a second if you really like her!)
- Common dating questions and concerns
- How to set boundaries during dates
- What to do at the end of and after a date
- How to navigate trickier or more specific scenarios, such as falling for a friend or a co-worker, or reconnecting with an ex

Dating women can be hot, hilarious and sometimes downright confusing, but it can also be one of the most affirming parts of your queer journey. So whether you're nervous, excited or somewhere in between, just know: you've got this. And we're going to unpack it all, together.

Is dating a woman different to dating a man?

The number one question I get asked on social media is: 'How is dating a woman different from dating a man?'

When you strip it back, queer women's hopes, desires, fears and needs around communication, vulnerability and emotional and physical attraction aren't so different from anyone else's.

What changes is how those pieces interact, the way connection feels, and how intensely it sometimes shows up when two women fall in love.

Aka, the *dynamic*.

When two women fall for each other, the emotional bond can feel incredibly strong, sometimes faster and deeper than you expect. Vulnerability tends to surface early, and with it comes a connection that's raw, real and intensely intimate.

That's not to say this kind of connection can't happen with men – it absolutely can – but many queer women (me included) will tell you that there's something different and magnetic in how quickly and intensely things tend to develop with another woman.

Part of this comes down to biology. Our bodies produce a hormone called oxytocin, sometimes nicknamed the 'bonding hormone', which plays a big role in emotional attachment. In addition to this, biologically speaking, women also tend to be more tuned in to things like tone of voice, facial expressions and subtle shifts in mood, which can make us more sensitive to emotional nuances in relationships and social interactions.

This emotional awareness means that in relationships between women there's often a high level of empathy and emotional responsiveness right from the start.

It can create a beautiful feedback loop: one person opens up, the other meets them (hopefully!) with care, and a strong sense of safety and intimacy starts to build. Interestingly, research shows that women in relationships with women tend to report more emotional support and mutual understanding than those in heterosexual pairings.

All of that can make the connection you're experiencing feel like a breath of fresh air, but it also means things can, at times, feel intense. When you're both tuned in emotionally, the highs are high, but any tension or conflict can feel more personal and exposing.

It's not always a bad thing, as long as you're aware of it.

Understanding the emotional dynamics at play – how biology, psychology and even gender roles influence connection – can help you approach your relationship with more clarity and compassion.

And just to be clear: this isn't about saying queer relationships are better or 'deeper' than straight ones. It's about recognising that when traditional gender roles fall away, the emotional landscape shifts too.

In heterosexual relationships, for example, there could be an argument that emotional labour often gets placed on one partner (usually the woman), while in queer relationships between women, there can be more shared responsibility and awareness around emotional needs.

So if you're stepping into a relationship with another woman, know that deep emotional connection is often part of the package. It's something to be cherished but also navigated with sensitivity. Because when two people show up with openness, honesty and mutual respect, what you create together can be truly rare and powerful.

What am I looking for?

Figuring out what you're looking for when you're new to dating women or putting yourself back out there (especially if it's been a while!) can feel daunting, and lots of questions might come up for you:

Am I attracted to someone more stereotypically 'femme'- or 'masculine'-presenting, or somewhere in between?

Should we like the same things or can we be different?

Do I want someone who's new to dating women too or someone very experienced to lead the way?

MY STORY

When I first decided I wanted to date women, I downloaded apps like Tinder and Bumble and began optimistically swiping on all types of girls. I had no idea what I was looking for, nor did I know what kind of woman I found attractive.

DATING

It felt a little bit like I was throwing everything at the wall and seeing what stuck – and (even though it might feel a bit impersonal), sometimes you have to approach dating in this way, especially at the start, so you can quickly learn what you do and don't like.

One of my first dates was with a beautiful Australian woman called Anna* who rocked up half an hour late. I was waiting for her in a Starbucks and when she finally arrived she sat down in front of me, reached across the table, chugged the remainder of my coffee, ate the cake from my plate and then proceeded to tell me that she hadn't been successful in finding a girlfriend yet because apparently she was quite 'dominant'. Needless to say, we didn't meet up again.

A wonderful first date I went on was with an Irish girl called Naoimh*. We went out for burgers and bowling and couldn't stop laughing. At the end of the date, we kissed, but the laughter continued in a very different way as we quickly realised we'd be much better suited as friends than lovers, but both agreeing that it was the most fun we'd had in a long time.

One of the more unusual dates I've been on was with a woman who lived merely a few streets away from me. We met up in the local pub. She arrived in sunglasses and a rugby sweatshirt and had I not asked her any questions I'm sure she would have stayed mute. It transpired that she worked in 'a government department' (which I believe was a cover for being a spy), as she gave limited information away about her life other than her interest in finance, history and potatoes. The conversation was very stunted and we parted ways after an hour, only for her to walk into a back alley and disappear. I never saw her again.

Dating different types of people can be a great way to learn about yourself and what you value and want (or perhaps don't want!) in a partner. It opens your mind, challenges your assumptions and helps you grow. But it also raises the question: how do you figure out your *type* and should you even have one in the first place? So let's get into that now.

How do I figure out my type?

Having a 'type' stirs up different reactions for different people. Some see it as helpful to be on the lookout for a certain type of person, and others will say it's best to keep your options open.

I personally believe that it's healthy to know what you like in another person, so long as it doesn't hold you back if someone outside of these parameters shows up, who you might be interested in.

I have always known what kind of woman I like based on who catches my eye from across a bar right the way through to who I think looks hot on the cinema screen. She's usually an older woman with long hair and a dark sense of humour, slightly jaded, always armed with a glass of wine and sporting a pair of sunglasses, like she's on the run from Interpol. (What can I say? The mystery is part of the charm.)

If you're new to figuring out your type and you're unsure where to start then I would recommend going for a drink/coffee/walk (whatever feels comfortable to you) with a variety of *very* different people. It won't take long for you to understand what turns you on and off.

For more insight, I asked some queer women how they navigate figuring out their type, or even if they believe in types at all:

QUEER VOICES

'I have key qualities, both physical and personality, that I look for in women. It was a matter of testing the waters with different people and seeing what matched the best.'

'I like to think I don't believe in types but my friends will constantly remind me that I have never dated someone under six feet tall.'

'I don't think types are a helpful concept for me, in the same way as I don't find labels super useful, either. If a "type" means a set of character traits rather than physical appearances then I can get more on board with that. I'm typically attracted to someone's open mind, emotional depth, and a sense of humour is always a winner, too!'

'I love femme-presenting women but I'm more attracted to someone's energy and look for deep connections. If she can command the room, stimulate me intellectually and make me laugh, I'm f*cked. Past relationships really helped guide me to what I actually desire . . . and don't.'

'I've always thought my type was mascs, but now that I've been out for several years, I'm starting to find femme girls more and more attractive. I think my attraction towards mascs, although very real, was a form of internalised homophobia. If I was only attracted to masc women, then it would be acceptable after dating men my whole life. Now I'm opening up to the fact that I'm attracted to more feminine women.'

'I think types are definitely a thing, but I also think that many of us are taught what our type "should" be, due to what we internalise about beauty standards and the like. So it's often worth asking the question, "Is this person my type, or is this just who I'm being told I should be attracted to?" I find that my types are defined by their personality and how they act more than their looks.'

Should I have a type or should I look for shared interests and values instead?

Building out a 'type' of person that you would like to date or potentially form a relationship with is an ever-changing process, because as we evolve and grow on our journey of understanding ourselves, naturally what we're looking for in another person (or people) is probably going to change.

My type isn't just limited to sunglasses and long hair (see above) but what *characteristics* that person embodies. I like people who are sarcastic, kind, open-minded and practical, so therefore this is the mental checklist in my head that someone would need to meet for there to be *any* level of attraction.

I personally think creating a checklist rather than a type is a fun way to approach dating, so long as you don't take it too seriously!

Looking at the qualities and values someone brings to the table is a good exercise in defining what's important to you, and in turn identifying the kind of people who might not be the right fit. This isn't to say that you should judge someone immediately – it's more of a way to check in with yourself to see if the connection you're part of aligns with who *you* are, and what *you* want.

I remember a conversation with a friend just before she started dating her now fiancée. She told me she created a non-negotiable list to guide her through the dating scene. It included the following:

- Must like roller coasters
- Must not like watching long Marvel movies
- Must like scary movies

It made me laugh so much that I started my own:

- Must be able to cook and appreciate food
- Must like being outdoors and getting muddy on a walk
- Must want to dance with me at a party

Try it, maybe with a friend. If nothing else, it's a fun game!

Should we have the same interests or do opposites really attract?

In my opinion it's healthy to have both similarities and differences when dating someone, so you can learn new things, grow and expand your mindset. It's also a healthy thing to enjoy activities and experiences *separately* so you're not always in each other's pockets (a dangerously common theme for women who date women).

The real bond that holds you together, though, goes beyond surface-level interests. It's rooted in the values you share and how much importance you place on certain activities, experiences and how you choose to spend your time.

Having a conversation around what someone is passionate about is a great way to uncover this. Try to go beyond talking about work, TV shows and everyday life. Really try to understand the lens through which the other person sees the world, so you can see if this is aligned with yours.

Some really great conversation starters would be:

- **'What are you excited about right now?'** – Maybe they're working on a project, travelling or volunteering somewhere.
- **'How do you feel about . . . ?'** – Try to keep this light-hearted, especially if you're on the first few dates, but getting their opinion on something that matters to you can be really telling and help you see if you view things in a similar light.
- **'What do you find funny?'** – Crack some jokes and see if they land! Does your energy align in this way and do you find the same things hilarious?

What you really need to uncover is how the time you spend together makes you feel. It won't be perfect all the time, but if you feel that they *get* you, then this is a really positive step.

Love language

Some people like to use the love languages framework outlined by Dr Gary Chapman in his 1992 book *The Five Love Languages: How to Express Heartfelt Commitment to Your Mate* to understand their partners more.

Although it's not a full read of how compatible you are with someone, I think it's a cute way to open up the conversation on how to start seeing another person and show up for them in the way they'd like to be cared for.

Below is a quick breakdown of Dr Chapman's 'Five Love Languages':

- **Words of affirmation** – Love is expressed through verbal compliments, appreciation, encouragement and kind words.

- Examples: 'I love you', 'You mean so much to me' or 'You did a great job'.
- **Acts of service** – Love is shown by doing things for your partner that make their life easier or more enjoyable.
- Examples: Cooking a meal, running errands or helping with chores.
- **Gifts** – Love is felt through the giving and receiving of thoughtful gifts.
- Examples: It's not about materialism but the thought and effort behind the gift.
- **Quality time** – Love is expressed by giving undivided attention and spending meaningful time together.
- Examples: Deep conversations, shared activities or just being fully present.
- **Physical touch** – Love is communicated through physical affection.
- Examples: Hugs, holding hands, cuddling or more intimate touch.

These tools can be conversation starters you can pull out on a date and they will likely offer you an insight into the person sitting in front of you, so give them a go!

What kind of relationship structure am I looking for?

Understanding the type of relationship structure or dynamic you'd like to enter into as a queer woman can sometimes be tricky. It involves an understanding of the type of person *you* are, *who* you would like to date and what qualities they embody.

Monogamous relationships are often the default starting point for many queer women, partly because they're the model most of us see reflected around us. They can offer a sense of clarity and emotional grounding as you're figuring out who you are, what you want and how you show up in a partnership. The focus on one person can make it easier to build trust, explore intimacy and develop your communication skills without navigating multiple dynamics at once. It doesn't mean the relationship is simpler – healthy monogamy still requires communication, boundaries and self-awareness – but it can feel more contained and therefore easier to understand as you're learning what you value in love and connection.

But while monogamy can be a fulfilling and grounding structure, it's not the only way queer people build relationships. Some find that once they understand the foundations of connection, trust, communication, emotional insight, they're curious about how those same skills might expand in different relationship models. That's where polyamory or open relationships come in: a kind of 'queer 2.0', where the core principles of monogamy are still essential but applied across more than one dynamic. It takes emotional intelligence, honesty and a strong sense of self, but if exploring multiple connections feels aligned with who you are, there's no reason to shy away from it, even if you're newly out and still discovering what you want.

I looked for solid stats on how many LGBTQ+ couples are polyamorous and it's tricky, because many studies focus on individuals, not couples, and definitions vary. But the picture that *does* emerge is interesting. In the 2023 OPEN survey of people practising non-monogamy, over half (57 per cent) identified as LGBTQIA+ (lesbian, gay, bisexual, transgender, queer or questioning, intersex, asexual, aromantic or agender, other) and 60 per cent of respondents self-identified as polyamorous. Rubel and Burleigh's 2020 study also estimates that between 0.6 per cent and 5 per cent of adults in the USA are polyamorous at a given time, with lifetime exposure somewhere between 2 per cent and 23 per cent, depending on how broadly you define polyamory. So yes, it's not quite mainstream (yet), but it's far from rare. And for queer people, it's clearly a visible and meaningful way of doing relationships.

My advice to anyone wishing to navigate polyamory is to talk to others who are already doing it, watch videos online and read books. Understand if it's something you'd like.

There's no shame in exploring it.

I asked queer women to share their experiences of engaging in either open relationships or polyamorous dynamics; their thoughts are below:

QUEER VOICES

'I've only really been in a couple of monogamous relationships. I've always known that a polyamorous lifestyle is what makes sense and what works for me. Multi-partner relationships have forced me to be more open with communication, to learn to trust my heart (and trust others!) and helped me understand and deal with jealousy. These are all important skills for existing in a society and I feel like a more understanding and compassionate person when I utilise them in other areas of socialisation.'

'I had an open relationship. It allowed me to explore after my divorce in a way that felt safe. It did end in tears, though, because one person decided they wanted exclusivity in the end and the other didn't want that with that person. Awks.'

'Yes. I thought I could have my cake and eat it too. In reality, jealousy is hard to manage and I just don't have the energy to be in a dynamic like that. I'm better off balancing other aspects of my life like family, friends, business and hobbies.'

'I have but I didn't enjoy it. I learned some people are poly and some people are not.'

'I've been in a polyamorous relationship. I think they can definitely work with a LOT of open communication. They are definitely not for everyone and I personally didn't love it at the time. But with the right people and being in the right mindset myself I could see it being wonderful to have different partners to satisfy different needs.'

Where to meet other queer women

So now you've figured out (albeit loosely) who you might be looking for in a room of people, but that leads us to the next burning question ... where the f*ck is that room? And where are all the queer women *actually* at?

One of the questions I get asked most often by women who are new to dating women is, 'Where do I find a woman to date?'

It's totally normal to feel nervous or even a bit overwhelmed by the idea of putting yourself out there – it can feel like stepping into the unknown, and that's scary! But nervous energy can actually be a sign that something exciting is about to happen.

Meeting new people, especially in a queer space, isn't just about finding a date – it's about opening the door to connection, community and maybe even the L word (no, not lesbian) . . . love.

So, instead of letting anxiety hold you back, try to see it as an opportunity to discover not just someone else, but more about yourself too.

Let's break down where you can meet queer women and how to lean into that exciting, sometimes nerve-wracking moment with confidence.

Online dating

This is one of the most obvious and popular routes into dating if you're a newly out or questioning queer woman. It offers you a chance to quite literally 'browse' the market, see who takes your fancy and make a move from the comfort of your own environment.

Dating apps are a wonderful tool for those looking to date fast, those who perhaps live outside of a city and wish to connect with others in different parts of the country and those who want to practise the art of online conversation and flirting.

My advice for anyone new to dating women and using apps is to lead with your personality and pick photographs of yourself that showcase what you love and who you are. Attracting women can be a very different ball game to attracting men. From speaking to people in my community, the common consensus is that women generally want to see other women laughing, having fun and sharing their hobbies, We're less interested in seeing six photos of you in a bikini staring blankly at the camera (some women might like this, but I'd question their motives if so).

Dating apps should be about having fun and seeing who you vibe with, so write something unique and interesting about yourself. It doesn't have to be wild – it can be as simple as what your favourite food is or where you love to travel. Showcase who you are and the right people will come back to you.

Opinions on the use of dating apps in the queer women community is divided, and although there are no specific stats to back this up, through my own experience and talking to friends in the community I know that some women swear by them and find great dates or even long-term partners, and some women refuse to use them at all.

I think it comes down to what type of person you are, and how you fall for someone. I used dating apps religiously in my 20s and had a lot of fun talking to people on there, but as I've gotten to know myself better and understand how I truly fall for a person, I've realised that they don't particularly serve me. It's not that I dislike them, it's just that the qualities I look for in a date are ones I can usually only find by interacting with someone in a real-world setting. I'm happy to have my mind changed, though, and sometimes after a few drinks (spurred on by my friends) I'll download them just to see what's going on.

But what I will say is that dating app algorithms will never be able to match how human connection works. The online space is very different to reality and online platforms lack the crucial elements needed for attraction, such as chemistry (which can only be found once in proximity to another person or people) and the art of connection (talking and bouncing off each other naturally).

I would definitely recommend dating apps to those who are newly out in the community to build confidence and understand yourself further, but I also recommend not passing by the connections in real life, as perhaps what you're looking for might be staring you right in the face already.

Parties and events

Real-life events are great places to meet other women. These might take the form of parties, networking events, Pride celebrations or more. The only challenging thing to consider is that most of these gatherings tend to happen in larger towns or cities, so if you live outside of these areas then you may have to travel in order to attend.

In London we have a super vibrant scene for queer women. No matter what age or vibe you're looking for, there are specific parties and networks. The best way to find out about these is through literally googling 'events for queer women in [fill in your location]' or searching on TikTok and Instagram.

Attending an event solo can definitely feel intimidating, but the queer community is, more often than not, incredibly welcoming and open to meeting new people. If you're nervous, bringing a plus-one can make a big difference, as someone you can bounce off socially as you both ease into the space and start making connections. Whether your plus-one is queer or an ally doesn't really matter; what counts is that you feel supported. And who knows, your friend might even discover something new about themselves along the way too!

It usually doesn't take long to find your people and start building confidence. Once you feel more comfortable, you'll naturally begin to expand your circle and that might also include chatting to people you're attracted to. The best approach is to go in with the intention of forming genuine, platonic connections and stay open to whatever else might unfold, without putting pressure on yourself or anyone else.

Friends

When you open up your world to meeting new people, you will soon find that you have new connections and build new friendships in the queer space. This is great because often when those friends have events, birthdays and parties you'll get an invite to them too, which means new network, new people, new possibilities.

One of the perks of meeting a potential date through a friend is that they often come somewhat 'pre-vetted'. (Though, a note of warning, the quality of that vetting can sometimes vary!) Still, it usually means you have a bit more context. You can ask questions, get a feel for who they are, and even learn a bit about their dating history, which can be surprisingly helpful.

That said, it's important not to approach friendships with the hidden agenda of scoping out their social circle for potential 'leads'. Instead, stay open to possibilities and approach new connections with genuine curiosity and kindness. Don't fixate on finding *someone*: focus instead on placing yourself in spaces that feel aligned with your energy and values. The right connections tend to grow naturally from there.

Groups

Similar to the parties and networking events above, there are also plenty of ways to get involved with groups, depending on your specific interests. Great examples of these would be interest groups like running and football, reading and book clubs, discussion groups, performance and improv/drag or even attending one-off events that interest you such as picnics or podcast recordings.

You can choose to attend more generalised groups for the LGBTQ+ community (which queer women will be at) such as LGBTQ+ sports clubs or even Pride networks at your place of work, or seek out more specialised groups in the lesbian/bi/queer space that are female (usually nonbinary and trans) inclusive.

I would personally recommend doing both. The benefit of this is that you are not only meeting potential people who you might like to date but a wide variety of people who *already* share common ground, so therefore you have something you can build on, whether it's romantic or just platonic, so the exercise in getting yourself out there isn't so pressurised.

Queer travel – groups for female, nonbinary and trans travellers

Another great way to meet people, especially if you love to travel, is through group trips designed specifically for queer women, trans and nonbinary travellers (like the ones that I host – check out my social media accounts, for more information).

As mentioned in chapter 3, travelling with a group creates a unique environment where bonds form quickly and deeply. Sharing new experiences, navigating unfamiliar places together and stepping outside your routine can lead to genuine connections, romantic or otherwise.

The goal isn't to go into these trips with the expectation of finding a partner, but rather to stay open to the possibilities of who you might meet along the way. These journeys are about exploration in every sense: new places, new people and new parts of yourself.

People are drawn to energy that's alive and authentic. So challenge yourself, uplift yourself and keep blooming into who you are becoming.

Don't chase the butterflies. Instead, plant your own beautiful meadow, and trust that the butterflies will find their way to you.

I asked my community of queer women how they approach dating and where they like to find connections. As you will see, the answers are extremely varied:

QUEER VOICES

'I've dated with Hinge, Bumble, through friends, and at social/athletic clubs intended for queer folks.'

'I have always found attending classes to be the best way to meet new people. Find a burlesque class, intro to drag, etc. I met my current partner at a queer self-defence class.'

'Any friendships or relationships that I've had, we met in real life at events or through friendship groups. I think it depends if you're looking for a romantic partner who has a specific interest – it's always a good idea to join a collective of ladies who like to do that specific thing!'

'I've actually met most of my long-term partners at work . . . Dating apps have never really led to anything significant for me. I think I'm more suited to organic, in-person connections that evolve into romance over time, when the feelings are mutual.'

'I prefer meeting romantic partners IRL. But so many amazing friendships sprung out of failed dating-app dates!'

'For me dating apps are basically slot machines for validation. One swipe and you're like, "Am I hot? Smart? Why don't they like me? I'm a good person!" Cue existential crisis over strangers you don't even know.'

'I try to go to organised things I see on Instagram. [They're] mainly London-based, which isn't great, but plan it well, go with a friend, watch your booze intake and smile!'

The F word

So you're just starting to find your feet with women. Perhaps you've attended a few events and figured out your type, or maybe you're open to exploring all opportunities, but what happens when it comes to communicating how you feel and the dreaded F word (no, not that one just yet): FLIRTING?

Let's be real, flirting can make even the most confident people nervous, especially when you're unsure of how your interest will be received. It's easy to freeze up, overthink or avoid making a move altogether. But here's the good news: flirting is a skill, not a mystery, and you *can* learn it.

In this section, we're going to unpack what it takes to be effortlessly seductive, hear from other queer women about how they flirt, and pick up some top tips along the way.

Instead of doing the classic gay girl thing and ignoring someone you're interested in for fear of rejection (yes, I've clocked you!), let's look at how you can actually start to feel confident and begin engaging with someone...

Watch others

This is a little secret of mine and I've been doing it for years. I'm not talking about intensely staring at strangers across a restaurant or bar – that'd be weird. What I mean is paying attention to movies, TV shows and social media to notice those subtle, effortlessly hot moves people make:

- The way someone tilts their neck = hot. I'll steal that.
- The way someone winks after they drop a funny line = hot. I'll steal that.
- The way someone touches (please make it consensual) the small of another person's back as they leave the bar = hot. I'll be using that.

This isn't to say that you should change your personality and become someone else, but to find the little things that you think you could copy and put your own spin on.

Seriously, try it. It's a game changer.

Get a wing woman or man

Nothing beats having back-up if you're going out to a party, bar or social event. Not only can you talk about how much you're absolutely shitting yourself with your mates, but you can also support each other by starting conversations with other people.

Finding a confident and funny wing person is a gift from the gods. Just remember not to drink too much with them – you don't want to look like a comedy act on tour (or maybe you do – it's definitely worked for me in the past).

Listen loudly

In his 2023 book *How to Know a Person*, David Brooks talks about the concept of really leaning into listening. Elaborate when you speak and don't fake it. If you're inspired by what the other person is saying, let your eyes light up in delight. If you're shocked by a funny story then let your mouth hang open a bit.

You're an interesting person, so let them see that. Don't stand there like a static baguette.

Physical closeness

When you find yourself leaning closer to someone or subtly mirroring their movements, it's not just in your head: your heart is actually communicating through its own electromagnetic signals. The heart produces an electromagnetic field about 5,000 times stronger than the brain's, and studies show that when people spend time close together, their heart rhythms can actually sync. This 'heart syncing' helps create emotional bonds and builds trust.

For queer women, whose flirting often happens through subtle, non-verbal cues, this physical closeness sends a powerful unspoken message of attraction. So the next time you're on a date try sitting next to her rather than across from her, lightly touch her arm or perhaps brush her hand as you're walking!

Eye contact and smiling

We all know the power of eye contact, but are you brave enough to let it linger for a split second longer than it should? That's the art of flirtation, baby. Don't stare but don't look away too soon. Couple it with a little smirk or a smile and my job here is done. The other person will know exactly what's going on if you can pull off this move.

Be funny (or at least try to be)

Everyone loves a good sense of humour and if you're naturally funny then you're already one step ahead.

Use your humour in small doses – be playful and tease them a little bit over something small and safe (like their drink choice or how much they might be complaining about the weather). The trick here is to keep it polite but a little bit sassy and playful.

Confidence is hot, but don't knock them down!

Drop a line

I'm not really into using scripted lines when I meet someone, but there's one a friend shared with me that never fails. The secret is having the confidence to deliver it smoothly.

'Have you ever slept with a woman before?'

If they say 'no' you just follow up with:

'Would you like to?'

It's cheeky, I know, but come back to me and say it hasn't worked, I dare you.

For me, there's one clear sign that I'm into someone as more than a friend, and it's not on the list above. Unfortunately, it's also way less subtle than I'd prefer: I start biting my lower lip.

I wish I could stop, but I simply can't. It's my brain's way of saying, *Yep, you like this person. Quit pretending.* Then again, there are worse giveaways, so if you get a lip bite from me ... just know, I think we'd be good together.

DATING

I was curious about how other women show their interest when they flirt, so I asked my community of queer women how they show attraction with the women they're into. Now *you* get to learn all their little moves, subtle tells and scandalous secrets:

QUEER VOICES

'I like good eye contact, little touches and using someone's name: it feels intimate and intentional. I also ask questions and make them laugh: humour and curiosity are my bag.'

'Never underestimate the power of a light touch and well-timed eye contact.'

'I naturally like to tease and be sarcastic!'

'I find that if I'm really attracted to someone, I naturally gravitate closer to them. So if I'm making a lot of eye contact and clumsily bumping into your personal space, I'm probably very into you!'

'Through eye contact, body language and leaning in. If I'm into you, I'm also going to show interest through conversation that goes beyond surface level. If I feel you're reciprocating, I may just come out and tell you that I'm into you!'

'If you want to kiss her, say, "I've been wanting to kiss you since [fill in the blank]." Don't stay silent. Say it! And if she's giving you eye contact, that's how you know.'

> **Don't stay silent. Say it!**

'If I'm feeling the vibe, I ask if I can get an eyelash off their cheek and kiss them while I'm there.'

'If I'm feeling cheeky, I say, "You've been on my mind since X [pick something silly or cute that they've done, which is a subtle tease]." If she laughs and looks at me, I'll lightly touch her hand and say, "Can I make you forget about it with a kiss?" Works every time.'

How do I know if she's into me or just being friendly?

This is one of the most common questions women ask, whether they're newly out or have been part of the community for some time. The line between friendship and something more can be subtle (and we'll unpack this further in chapter 7) but there are a few clues that might reveal if she's interested in you romantically.

That said, context really matters. For example, if the person you like is neurodivergent, the signs they show might look different from those of someone who is neurotypical.

Generally speaking, though, if you can check off a few of the following signs, you're already halfway there!

Verbal clues

Interest

If a woman is asking you a lot of questions about yourself, and she's actually *listening* to your answers, then there's already a level of interest there.

Psychologists point out that asking questions (especially follow-ups) signals curiosity: it shows someone wants to understand you and is investing attention in you. On dates, people who ask more follow-up questions tend to be liked more by their partner and are more likely to get asked out again.

If the conversation goes deeper than 'What do you do for work?' – if it dives into *why* you like something, your family, your past relationships or beliefs – that's a clue she's trying to see you more fully, not just casually.

Of course be mindful of boundaries here, though. Nobody wants to be interviewed over an after-work beer!

Nervous energy

When we're nervous we tend to talk shit. Everyone does it. It's especially bad if you're talking to someone attractive and you forget what your thread of conversation is halfway through.

Psychology gives us some clues about why this happens. Nervousness triggers the body's stress response (fight-or-flight), which produces adrenaline and increases arousal. That excess energy often needs an outlet, and talking becomes one, almost like a safety valve. When words come out, they distract the mind from internal tension and physical symptoms of nervousness.

Also, socially, we humans seek connection and reassurance. When you're with someone attractive, you subconsciously want them to like you. Overtalking, explaining yourself, filling silences – these are ways to reduce uncertainty, signal friendliness and test if you're safe.

So when you notice someone being overly chatty around you, jumping between topics and darting off the main thread, it might feel chaotic but it can also be a clear sign they're nervous *and* interested.

Remembering details

If you've had a few interactions with this person and they remember little details about you – your coffee order, where you're going on holiday, how you wear your hair or what you've watched on Netflix recently – that person is probably digging you.

There's more than just 'chance' behind those little moments of remembering, though. Psychology tells us that remembering romantic details is closely tied to how much someone cares, how attuned they are and how much emotional weight we assign to our early connections.

Studies also show that women generally have a better memory for romantic relationship events than men, especially when it comes to recalling fine details from dates or meaningful shared moments. In one study, 'Gender differences in romantic relationship memories: who remembers? Who cares?' (great title) women in relationships with men reported more vivid and detailed memories of their relationship events, and these memories correlated with higher relationship well-being.

For queer women, those moments of attention can feel especially meaningful, because sometimes your social spaces have taught you that your queer identity, your dating life or your emotional self are less visible than heteronormative narratives. So when someone listens, remembers or acts on those small details, it signals presence, care and respect. It tells you: 'I see *you*. I'm paying attention beyond the surface.'

Compliments

Women love to compliment other women, but if the person you're interested in is dishing out the compliments left, right and centre, then they're literally noticing *everything* about you – your outfit, the way you speak, how you smile, even how your energy feels.

There's also some psychology behind this. Research shows that women tend to be more attuned to detail and emotional nuance than men, especially in social and romantic settings. Studies have found that women are generally better at interpreting and recalling emotionally relevant cues, such as what someone said, how they looked or even the tone in which something was expressed.

Other studies interestingly show that women often outperform men in facial and visual memory tasks, which helps explain why they're more likely to notice and remember these little things.

So, if a woman is noticing and naming all the things she appreciates about you, from your shoes to your laugh, chances are it's not casual. Compliments are often a soft way of signalling attraction, especially in queer spaces where lines between friendship and flirting can blur. If she's constantly finding reasons to praise or highlight you, she's likely feeling more than just friendly vibes.

Laughter

You're either very funny or you're not *that* funny and the other person digs it. Either way it's a great sign. True smiles and genuine laughter are hard to fake and they light up the brain's reward system. Neuroscience even shows us that laughter releases endorphins which not only make us feel good but also builds social bonds and trust.

For queer women, who often navigate relationships where emotional intimacy is especially valued, shared laughter can be a powerful way to break down barriers and signal safety and attraction. It's a non-verbal way of saying 'I like being around you' and 'I feel comfortable enough to let my guard down.' So while laughter alone isn't a guaranteed sign of attraction, making someone light up like that definitely means you're halfway there.

Teasing

Is she mimicking your voice, playfully teasing you, or even challenging you in a light-hearted game of who's 'right' or 'wrong'? These are classic signs she's interested in more than just friendship. Psychologically, teasing is a form of flirtation that signals closeness and affection while testing boundaries in a safe, playful way.

For queer women, who often value emotional connection and nuanced communication, this kind of playful banter can create a fun, intimate space where attraction grows naturally.

Teasing helps build rapport and shows confidence. It's a way of saying 'I'm comfortable enough with you to joke around, and I want you to notice me.' It also activates the brain's reward centres, releasing dopamine and making interactions feel exciting and engaging. So if your date is teasing you, it's not just about the laughs: it's her way of signalling interest and testing chemistry.

Body language

Learning how to read the body language of another person is an art in itself, but learning how to read another woman is a skill that you *need* to know. Not only is it hot to play around with this but it also allows you to garner valuable insights into how the other person feels without needing to ask (especially helpful if you haven't yet defined what this thing 'is' between the two of you).

Playing with hair and/or fiddling with jewellery and rings

This isn't just a nervous habit: it's a classic sign of attraction. Psychologically, this behaviour is a form of *preening*, something we share with animals like peacocks who fluff their feathers to look their best for a potential mate. For women, including queer women on dates, these subtle actions are subconscious ways of signalling interest and care about how they're perceived.

Preening helps draw attention to features they want you to notice and shows they're invested in the interaction. It's a non-verbal flirtation, communicating 'I want to look good for you' without saying a word.

The eyebrow flash

This one is incredibly quick and subtle, so you'll need to be on the lookout for it, but when you enter the room or she sees you for the first time, a key sign of attraction is a quick lift and drop of the eyebrows, known as the 'eyebrow flash'. Research suggests that eyebrow flashes can foster connection by signalling friendliness and an openness to connect, encouraging mutual engagement.

Pheromones

Throwing her head back or tilting her neck to one side to expose her neck is a subtle but powerful sign of attraction. For many women, this gesture happens naturally because the neck is a sensitive area rich in pheromone release, which plays a key role in subconscious attraction cues. Some studies indicate that we emit and respond to subtle chemical cues – not fully like classic animal pheromones, but enough to affect mood, attraction and social connection

By exposing the neck, women may be instinctively inviting connection, drawing attention to an intimate and vulnerable part of their body. When you notice a woman tilting her neck or throwing her head back during a conversation or glance, it's often her body's way of signalling interest and openness, even before words come into play.

Breathing in deeply

Breathing in deeply is a subtle but telling sign of attraction. When someone is nervous or excited, the body naturally reacts by increasing heart rate, and taking a deep breath helps regulate these physical responses, calming the nervous system and slowing the heart rate.

So if she's talking faster than usual or taking more noticeable breaths, it's a good sign you've stirred something in her – a mix of nervous energy and excitement.

Eye contact

Eye contact is one of the most powerful nonverbal cues in attraction. Holding someone's gaze for three seconds or more can create a spark of sexual tension and signal interest. When she glances your way in a group setting to check if you're laughing at the same joke or holds your gaze just a bit longer than usual, it's often a sign she's paying extra attention to you.

Psychologically, eye contact activates the brain's social and reward centres, releasing dopamine and oxytocin, which deepen feelings of connection and attraction. This is especially meaningful in queer female relationships, where emotional and physical intimacy are often closely intertwined.

That said, it's important to remember that for some people, especially those who are nervous, shy or neurodivergent, direct eye contact can be challenging or uncomfortable. So, a lack of prolonged eye contact doesn't necessarily mean disinterest. Context matters.

The triangle

When people feel attracted to someone, their gaze often follows a distinctive pattern called the 'triangular gaze'. This means their eyes move from one eye to the other, then down to the lips, and back up again, forming an unconscious triangle on your face. This subtle eye movement usually signals that their mind is either subconsciously, or sometimes consciously, imagining what it might be like to kiss you.

Psychologically, this pattern happens because the eyes and lips are key areas involved in intimate connection and communication. The triangular gaze is a quiet but unmistakable invitation, a dance of the eyes that says 'I'm interested' without a single word being spoken.

Light touch

Does she often touch your arm when you laugh, play with your hair or go in for a hug? If it's light and playful, that can definitely be a sign she's into you.

Psychologically, touch is one of the most powerful ways humans communicate affection and attraction. Light, casual touches release oxytocin, which helps build connection and trust between people.

In romantic contexts, light touch also signals comfort and interest without words. For women, who often prioritise emotional intimacy, these small physical gestures are a way of saying 'I want to be closer to you' in a way that feels natural and spontaneous.

That said, there's an important boundary here: no one likes feeling like they're being 'petted' or touched without consent. It's crucial to respect personal space and read the room, especially early on. When done right, these touches should feel like playful invitations to deeper connection, not pressure.

Use your voice

Reading body language and picking up on signs can definitely give you clues about someone's interest. But if you want complete clarity, better than all the subtle hints and signals, the easiest (but yes, often scariest) way is just to ask.

Putting your feelings out there might feel vulnerable, but it's the surest way to know where you stand.

If they're into you, great! If not, you save yourself the time and emotional energy spent guessing.

At the end of the day, open communication is the foundation of any meaningful connection, so don't be afraid to be honest and direct.

Going on your first date

Now let's look at what happens when we shift from flirting to something more. Perhaps you've engaged in a dance of eye contact for a few weeks and maybe you want to kick it up a notch and see where things go.

Let's walk through how you can do this, step by step (and still be smooth).

Should I tell them I'm new to dating women?

Let's start with a common question: if you're going on your first date with a woman, are you expected to tell them it's your first time? Is there some kind of unwritten rule in the queer community around this?

The short answer? No, you don't owe anyone your dating history. There's no 'official' expectation that you need to disclose that it's your first time dating a woman. You get to choose what you share, and when, based entirely on what feels right for you.

That said, I personally think honesty is the best policy. So, if you *do* feel comfortable sharing, I'd encourage it, not as an obligation, but as an act of vulnerability.

Vulnerability, when expressed with intention, is incredibly powerful. It helps build trust, lowers emotional walls and allows for real connection. And if the person you're on a date with is kind and emotionally mature, they won't see it as a red flag or something awkward – quite the opposite. They'll likely feel honoured that you've shared something personal, and it might even soften their view of you.

It *can* feel daunting if you feel like the other person has more experience than you. But try not to frame it like a confession. You're not 'admitting' to a crime, you're just sharing a bit of context. A simple, casual 'Just so you know, this is my first date with a woman' is more than enough. Think of it as a friendly FYI, not a dramatic reveal.

And remember, no one is an expert at something they've never done before. That includes dating. Plenty of women who've been dating other women for years still feel unsure or awkward at times.

Think back to when you were little and couldn't do something that now feels second nature, like tying your shoes or brushing your teeth. I vividly remember telling my mum, at age five, 'I'm not going to school because I don't know how to read.' And she calmly replied, 'That's exactly *why* you're going.'

When we're inexperienced, and it feels like everyone else is already miles ahead, it's easy to get overwhelmed. But that doesn't mean you shouldn't start.

How do I ask someone out on a date?

Asking someone out, whether it's for a coffee, a walk, a drink or a dinner date, can feel terrifying, no matter your gender. But it can be especially nerve-wracking if you're a woman who's new to dating other women.

What's important to remember is that the outcome, whether they say yes or no, is not a reflection of your worth. It's simply about where *they* are, at that moment. Their response is about their feelings, their timing and their circumstances, not a judgement of you.

It's easy to tie our self-worth to external validation, but here's the irony: the more you put yourself out there, follow your instincts and take those small, brave steps, the more confident, magnetic and at ease you'll start to feel. Showing up authentically is what makes you attractive, not being 'picked' by someone else.

Here are my top tips for asking someone out in a way that feels confident, clear and grounded.

Lay out your cards on the table with politeness and planning

As I've gotten older, I like to put my cards on the table early on in the dating process. If I like someone, I let my intentions be known. I'd rather care deeply about someone and get rejected than pretend that I don't care at all, to protect my ego.

Having said this, it's also important not to dive in straight away and scare off the other person. It's a delicate balancing act.

Ways to do it:

- 'Would you like to grab a coffee sometime?'
- 'I'd love to hear some more about X. Maybe you can tell me about it over a drink?'
- 'I love X activity – have you been to Y? We should totally check it out.'

The key here is for your invitation to sound *friendly* and *safe*. Don't be overbearing with 'So are you free tomorrow for a drink?' Nobody likes pressure. Keep it fun and playful yet communicative.

The only exception to this rule is if you're both on the same page and already heavily flirting. Sometimes assertiveness can be integrated into the conversation and a direct line like 'So when are we gonna do this?' can be hot. It's all about context!

- **Set a challenge** – If they've mentioned that they're good at a certain activity (perhaps bowling) then take this as a sign to challenge them to it. You've already got an activity on the table that you know they enjoy, so let them feel like you see them and give them a chance to showcase their skills!
- **Don't spend too long talking before you meet up** – If you're using a dating app and you've had some back-and-forth conversations and the vibe is good, arrange a date! The energy someone gives in person is often very different to the written word, so do a vibe check. There's nothing worse than spending all your time and effort talking to someone only to meet them and realise you don't have chemistry.
- **Don't invite your friends (unless you want to keep it casual)** – As tempting as it can be to ask someone to join you at a group activity,

it could be misinterpreted as a friend date, so if you're serious about getting to know someone without distractions then carve out the time to focus your energy on them. The only exception is if you've already had some chat and want to test the vibe in a more casual setting, like inviting your date to a picnic, a class or a house party. Having other people around can take the pressure off but just make sure there's enough of a crowd so it doesn't get awkward. You want a party of at least four people – not just you, your date and one random friend stuck in the middle feeling like a third wheel.
- **Be confident with it** – Don't set expectations on whether they will accept the invitation or not. Make your intentions known, ask the question, then put your phone down and do something else. Approach the situation with the mindset of: *It would be nice to get to know this person some more so let's see if it's reciprocal. If not then it's their loss but the ball is in their court now.* More often than not, they will likely pick up on that energy and it will work in your favour.

Where can we go and how can I make the date memorable?

When I was dating in my 20s, I had a go-to table at a Mexican bar in Soho. It had small plates, great cocktails plus a foosball table and games area, which was a total winner with the girls. I was so consistent with taking dates there, the staff would automatically reserve 'my table' when I booked.

It was all going brilliantly, until it wasn't.

Eventually, some of my old dates started showing up at the same bar *with their new dates*, and before I knew it, the whole basement had become this unofficial queer dating hub – a sea of exes, almosts and future maybes. Let's just say it got a little *too* interconnected, and I was low-key relieved when the bar eventually shut down.

The moral of the story? A great date spot is memorable, relaxed and gives you both something to do *other* than stare into each other's eyes. It's not necessarily about how cool the venue is – it's about finding a place that reflects something about you and gives your date a glimpse into your world. That could be:

- A comedy night (laughing is a great ice-breaker)
- A queer poetry or spoken word event
- A plant shop, IKEA or a garden centre (yes, a plant aisle has done wonders for some lesbians I know)
- A wine-tasting session, ceramic class or second-hand bookshop crawl
- A walk followed by hot chocolate in a good dog-spotting location

Ask yourself: *What do we both enjoy?* Are you both into Japanese food? Indie gigs? Roller skating? The more natural and fun the activity feels, the easier it'll be to relax, even if there's no romantic spark in the end.

One more thing: try to avoid one-off or non-flexible events (e.g. a gig on a single date) for a first meet-up. People are busy, and offering options like 'Hey, this exhibition is on all month, would you want to go sometime next week?' is more considerate and low-pressure.

I asked my community of queer women to suggest some great date ideas, so that you have some inspiration:

QUEER VOICES

'For a first date, I love a coffee and a walk in the park. It's such a low-pressure atmosphere and who doesn't need to get outside for some fresh air?'

'One of my favourite (especially first) date ideas is picking a movie you both love, putting it on and talking through it. It's instantly disarming to have something you both find familiar and comforting to take the pressure off. No awkward silences when the movie is there!'

'A simple craft activity is always fun – something easy and not too intimidating. A park hang with a picnic. Don't go to the movies – you want to be able to talk to the person and get to know them!'

'Vineyard, spa, musical cat cafes (yes, that's a real thing), plant shops, vinyl stores, farmers' markets, film events, etc.'

'Personally, I love a bit of indoor rock climbing (harnesses . . . ahem!) because nothing builds trust more than hanging off a rope from a great height!'

'Nature walks, poetry nights, live music or art galleries. Anywhere you can talk, connect and share an experience.'

Do something you both love.

'Sporty dates, such as going to the driving range or playing mini golf, are a great date idea as they put less of the pressure on the other person and more on concentrating on the activity/sport you're doing, which can be a great way to see if there's any chemistry, particularly on a sober date.'

'I love coffee shops for first meetings so you can keep it short if it's not going well.'

'Ask them what their favourite food is and take them somewhere that serves it. A new experience, from street tacos to Middle Eastern delights!'

'I love an escape room, bowling or a long walk somewhere. Dinner and bars are great but very pressured. Do something you both love.'

How do I make sure I feel safe on a date with a woman?

Now, let's get to the part that might sound boring, but really matters, especially for anyone who's about to go on their first-ever date with a woman.

When you're new to queer dating, a big unspoken question is: 'Is there anywhere I shouldn't go? Are some places safer or more comfortable than others?'

The truth is, yes, the environment can make a huge difference, especially when you're still finding your footing. While most larger cities have a strong culture of queer visibility and inclusion, there are still some places where public displays of affection (PDA) between women (or visibly queer people) can draw unwanted attention. So while you *shouldn't* have to think about these things, sometimes it's helpful to plan ahead.

Here's how to make sure you feel safe, seen and comfortable on your date:

Choose a queer-friendly or visibly inclusive venue
You don't need to hit up a full-on gay bar, but somewhere that regularly hosts queer events, has inclusive signage or is located in a progressive area can help you relax. Cafes, bars or event spaces that fly a rainbow or trans flag in the window are a quiet but clear signal that the space *gets it*.

Avoid places where you might feel watched or judged
Your local pub may serve great pints, but if Old Jimmy-Jim-Jim in the corner is going to glare every time you laugh too loud or hold hands, it's not the vibe you need. Trust your gut: if a space feels weird, don't second-guess yourself. It's not about hiding – it's about protecting your peace.

Check the vibe beforehand
Use online reviews, Instagram tags or even ask friends if they've been to a spot before. You can also search for local queer-run businesses or spaces – many cities now have directories that make this easy.

Build in an exit strategy
Especially for first dates, meet somewhere public and ideally during the day or early evening. If it doesn't go well or you feel uncomfortable, you want to be able to leave easily and safely.

Common dating questions and concerns

Now that you've picked a venue or an activity, let's dig right into how to make your date special and memorable. Here are some common questions that come up for queer women, before, during and even after that first initial meet-up.

'What do I wear?'

I think it's time that I let you guys in on a little secret. Back in 2015 I purchased a pair of black, high-waisted disco pants and wore them on a night out. I'm not in the habit of complimenting myself but I've never received so much attention in my life.

I decided to test the theory of my 'lucky pants' at future events and dates and strangely every time I put them on my legs it happened again, and again – and again.

These disco pants are head-turners. Ten years on and I'm still wheeling them out of the closet, because I know they work. They're not in fashion (in fact I don't think you can even buy them in stores any more) and nor are they particularly comfortable but they work a *charm*.

My advice to you is to find your equivalent of these pants. Something that works for your body type and makes you feel confident! It doesn't need to be Lycra or leather or some crazy material but the key here is that it *compliments* you and the vibe you're looking to put out on the date.

Are you particularly into gardening or nature? Maybe you should integrate some floral patterns into your date outfit. Do you really resonate with a certain brand that's colourful and happy to match your personality? Throw on some colour!

Make sure your *external* is aligned with your *internal* and I promise you that your confidence will shine through.

*Also side note: don't be concerned if your date shows up wearing the same T-shirt/jeans/dress as you. It won't be the first time and it certainly won't be the last. It's one of the quirks of dating women – just laugh it off!

'What the f*ck should we talk about?'

Let's be honest, dating is nerve-wracking. It doesn't matter how old you are, how you identify or how confident you normally feel. When you're sitting across from someone you fancy, trying not to sweat through your top, being *yourself* suddenly feels like a mythical concept.

That's why it helps to keep things playful. Dating should feel more like a fun exchange between two curious people than a serious job interview. A little lightness, humour and curiosity can go a long way, not just to ease the nerves, but to build real connection.

When you ask playful, interesting questions, you're not only making your date feel good, but you're also giving them a chance to show up as their most open, relaxed self. And when that happens, the energy between you starts to build in a natural, joyful way.

So instead of defaulting to small talk or diving straight into heavy topics like work, family or *how many kids they want*, keep it light at the start. Let the deeper stuff come naturally as the vibe grows.

Here are some conversation starters that are fun, unexpected and *way* more revealing than asking someone what they do for work. They'll also give you a genuine insight into the person sitting across from you, and maybe even set you up perfectly for date number two.

- **'What are your top three cuisines?'** – Now you know where to take them for date number two if it works out.
- **'What are you listening to at the moment?'** – Now you can get an insight into what they listen to and if this aligns with your music taste, plus you can curate the playlist for your next date!
- **'What do you think the story is with the couple/friends/person over there?'** – Now you can see how weird/creative/funny they are based on what they make up.
- **'What would your death row meal be?'** – Now you can see how good they are at thinking on the spot and also go on to ask them why they have picked certain items, to dig deeper into their personality.
- **'Do you think pineapple belongs on pizza?'** – Now you know if they're a psychopath or not. Definitely ask this question if they're Italian, by the way – you'll be in bed from the sexual tension/aggression in no time!

Aside from the conversation starters above you can also ask practical questions about their career aspirations, personal projects, family and dating history. Make sure not to go too heavy with this, though – your date shouldn't feel like they're on a job interview where you're mapping out a five-year plan for them over tapas.

How to set boundaries during dates

Let's talk about boundaries, because when someone crosses one, it feels awful. That's your emotional alarm system doing its job, waving its little red flag and saying, 'Nope, not OK.' Maybe they've asked something too personal too soon, overshared in a way that makes you squirm or said something that just doesn't sit right.

That's why naming your boundaries clearly and kindly, especially on a date, can be a total game changer. And no, it doesn't have to be awkward or confrontational. It can actually feel *really* empowering to say something like, 'Hey, I'm not super comfortable chatting about that just yet, maybe another time?' It sets the tone, protects your space and gives the other person a better idea of how to meet you where you're at.

Remember, everyone comes into dating with a different sense of what's 'normal', and what feels like casual chat for one person might feel way too deep or personal for someone else. So instead of shutting the conversation down with a bark or a big dramatic moment, just name it gently, keep it breezy and move on.

You get to be honest *and* stay connected – that's the sweet spot.

Who pays the bill?

This is a very valid question and one that I'm going to answer in the simplest terms. If you picked the place and it's more expensive than a usual restaurant/experience or activity, then in my opinion you should pay – and vice versa. If the experience is a mutual decision or you're feeling at all like you might not want to meet up again with this person, then split the bill. There is nothing worse than feeling in debt to someone you don't want to see again, but if you do want to see them again, then at least you've balanced each other out for the next time.

My ultimate top tip is to make sure you've remembered your cards, your pin or have access to pay on your phone. Don't embarrass yourself by not being able to pick up your share of the tab and making your date feel like a parent.

What do I do at the end of the date?

So you're on a first date with a woman and things have gone well. You leave the bar/activity/place of interest and walk towards the bus stop/tube/car park [insert your own method of transport here depending on where you live in the world]. You notice that your date is starting to look a little anxious and is shuffling their feet. The first thought going through your head is, *Oh god, do they want to kiss me or run away, or do I want to kiss them or do I want to run away?*

> **A sexy little bit of neuroscience for you . . .**
>
> Anxiety and sexual tension are often two sides of the same coin because they share many of the same neurochemicals that trigger similar physical and emotional reactions. When we're attracted to someone or feeling that spark of desire, our bodies release a cocktail of chemicals like adrenaline, dopamine, oxytocin, kisspeptin and norepinephrine. These neurochemicals activate the brain's reward and pleasure centres, making the situation feel thrilling, exciting and deeply engaging.
>
> At the same time, anxiety releases adrenaline and cortisol, hormones designed to put us on high alert in stressful situations. This heightened state can produce physical symptoms like a racing heart, sweaty palms and shortness of breath – the very same sensations we often interpret as 'butterflies' in the stomach during moments of attraction.
>
> Because of this overlap, our brains can blur the lines between fear and excitement. The neurochemical response to nervousness and sexual arousal is so similar that one can easily be mistaken for the other. A fascinating example of this is the 'misattribution of arousal' phenomenon, where people experiencing physiological

> arousal from fear or exercise might misinterpret it as attraction if presented with the right context.
>
> Even studies on people who have been 'fake kidnapped' or held hostage reveal that their heart racing and adrenaline surges mirror the same biochemical reactions that occur when someone experiences romantic or sexual excitement.
>
> The key difference between anxiety and sexual tension, then, is context: the brain's interpretation of these sensations is shaped by the situation and our perception of safety.
>
> So, that nervous energy you feel on a date? It could actually be your body's way of signalling that something exciting is happening, and it's completely normal to feel both exhilarated and on edge at the same time.

Basically, don't stress if you can't quite figure out why they're shuffling their feet at the end of a date. People are complicated, and chances are, they might not even fully understand their own feelings yet.

The easiest way to know if someone wants to kiss you? Just ask. Consent is sexy, and a simple line like 'I'd really love to kiss you' can be the perfect way to kick off a great make-out session.

And if the answer is no, don't be discouraged. There are plenty of reasons why someone might hold back: they might not feel the same way (better to know), they might be shy and prefer to wait until you're out of sight of others (totally valid, I'm not big on PDA myself) or maybe they just demolished a huge garlic bread and aren't exactly kiss-ready (also guilty as charged on that one).

Just read the vibe, check for consent and make your move if it feels right. Remember, kissing at the end of a date isn't a rule – it can sometimes be even more meaningful if you build up to it.

What if I'd like to see them again?

Much like initially asking someone out on a date, asking to see someone again can be daunting, especially if you're not too sure how the other person felt it went.

Usually you can pick up a vibe and hopefully your date will communicate how they feel while you're together, but just be prepared that this energy might shift once they've had time to reflect. Hopefully the sentiment will be shared, but it's always good to allow others the chance to breathe and take a beat to see if it's something they also want to pursue.

You could follow up the date with a simple message that reads: 'It was really lovely to hang out tonight, I'd love to do X [insert something meaningful here such as grabbing a coffee, going for a walk, seeing some comedy] again, so let me know if you're down!'

Equally you might not want to have a second date with the person and need to let them down in a gentle way. In this situation, you could share a message that reads along the lines of: 'I had a really nice time tonight. I'm not sure I'm feeling things beyond being friends though, so I just wanted to be transparent – but you're really lovely and I'd love to hang out again some time if you're up for it!' This way, the other person leaves the interaction feeling valued and less disheartened. But remember to only say you'd like to hang out if you genuinely have that intention, otherwise it's OK not to!

Specific situations

If you're new to dating women or starting to explore for the first time, you might have some more specific questions relating to the situation you find yourself in, so let's unpack these:

'I think I'm in love with my best friend'

It's a classic dilemma: should you tell them and risk the friendship, or keep it to yourself and wonder forever?

If you find yourself in this situation, I believe it's important to ask yourself a few key questions first:

1. **Is this really about them or is this about a longing for closeness with someone who understands and sees you?** – Our friends will always feel like safe spaces, as we have an established bond with them. If you're new to queer dating it could be to do with wanting a safety blanket, or it could be genuine attraction and romance. This is the first thing you need to figure out. I would recommend writing down the qualities that your friend brings and then seeking out connections with others who also embody those qualities, so you can weigh up how you feel in a new situation with someone different. Remember, it won't initially feel the same because you don't have that established bond, but it's an exercise in feeling out if it's specific to *them* or if it's coming from a need in *you*.
2. **Are you willing to risk the friendship if you're honest with them and they don't feel the same way about you?** – Offering up honesty about romantic feelings with someone can go both ways, depending on the strength and longevity of your friendship. I've known people to share their feelings with friends and they've ended up in happy relationships with each other; friends who couldn't get over the awkwardness of the dynamic changing and moved away from each other; and friends who've simply responded by saying, 'No, you don't fancy me – behave yourself!' and helped the other person to get over their feelings and direct them towards a new person, thus keeping their friendship intact. All of it comes with a risk, but if you feel that being honest is the only way forward then I encourage you to follow your intuition.
3. **Can you test the waters before you commit to splurging your feelings?** – If you have a feeling that your friend might be interested in you romantically, it's helpful to get some clarity before taking things further. I encourage you to look out for signs of attraction and then consider whether your feelings might be returned, if you're feeling nervous.

Crushes on friends can be complicated, but the best relationships often start with friendship. If you're already friends, in my opinion, you're already halfway to something great. Check out chapter 7 for much more information on navigating this grey area of love.

'I have a crush on my co-worker'

Having a crush on a co-worker is pretty common no matter your sexual orientation. However, speaking from experience with a few crushes on women at work over the years, here's some advice I can share:

- Flirting in an office environment is hot and feels taboo, so go for it! Just don't use the company's instant messaging systems or have your co-workers catch you in the act. People are often jealous of dynamics and this can cause unnecessary drama in the workplace. Stick to flirting on your personal platforms and reduce the length of your eye contact when you're around other people.
- Ask the person to lunch or after-work drinks and make it known that you'd like it to be only the *two* of you together. It can be tempting to include others in plans to pad things out or make it more casual, but sometimes you just have to rip off the plaster and go for broke – at least then you'll get your answer!
- Be careful who you tell. It might be tempting to share that you've got a little office fling happening but remember that other people might not want to hear about it, they might feel awkward or they might not agree with your choices. Keep it on the down-low and then when one of you leaves you can make it more public.
- If you're going to date them, make sure that they're not in charge of your pay. This creates an immediate power imbalance and if things don't end well between you, you're playing with fire. The only exception to this would be if either you or the other person has handed in their resignation or is moving to a different part of the business.

Many people I know have met their partners at work. It's a great way to get to know someone naturally over time. You see how they handle all kinds of situations, and honestly, it's pretty attractive to watch them in their element, taking charge. Just be sure not to get yourself fired in the process!

'Can I be in a long-distance relationship?'

I recently read a story about a queer woman called Meg Stone who sailed from Canada to Russia to collect her long-distance girlfriend Elena Ivanova so they could be together (I'll just let that sink in for a second). Due to their respective situations it was hard for them to find a country to settle in, so they have been living together at sea for many years. At the time of writing this, they are currently making a last-ditch effort to settle somewhere in Europe so they can build a home together permanently. Now that's one *heck* of an inspiring story of long-distance love (albeit in this case a forced separation), highlighting the extreme lengths queer women will go to, to be together.

It seems that long-distance relationships don't faze queer women. I don't know whether it's our inner romantic thinking that love is borderless or whether we've just been through so many other hurdles in our life that mileage isn't an issue, but either way, it's pretty common to find pairs of women who are racking up the air/land/nautical miles to be together.

Here are some top tips to consider if you are currently navigating or considering navigating a long-distance relationship:

- Find unique ways to connect with your partner, away from just voice messages and phone calls. You could try watching a movie together using the sharing feature on Netflix, spending time together on Facetime as you cook or hosting an online games evening. Finding different ways to connect and have 'virtual dates' will keep things interesting.
- Make sure that the travel is even and as fair as possible. Obviously this is down to each person's unique financial situation, but you don't want to end up in a place where one person is doing all of the legwork and the other is sitting back. It should be a shared effort.
- Always keep something to look forward to, whether it's a visit, a trip or simply talking about future times when you can be together again. Holding on to hope during times apart is crucial and making plans for when the distance is less helps keep that hope alive.

- Get support for your own mental health. Keep yourself busy with your own social life, activities, career and goals. It's important to have a full life outside of your partnership, especially if you're living apart. It might also be worth talking to a therapist about how you feel so you can be fully supported during this time.

Long-distance relationships take a lot of effort, trust, communication and boundary setting to work, but if you are able to come together and talk openly and honestly about your feelings and keep the relationship strong, then there's no reason why they can't work.

Who knows, maybe you'll buy your own boat and sail across the world for someone – queer women aren't afraid of making the effort!

'Should I get back with my ex or am I opening myself up for trouble?'

The tight-knit nature of the sapphic community can be a bit baffling to outsiders or those who are new in the space. Dating another woman means that a lot of the usual 'social norms' don't really apply. We're friends with exes, encourage our friends to date our exes, go on double dates with our new girlfriends and their ex-partners – it's all just a bit of a mash-up.

The reason for this is predominantly that while having a romantic relationship with another woman, we usually build an incredibly strong foundation for a friendship alongside it too.

This of course isn't the case for everyone, and many queer women that I know choose to move on entirely from the connection. But for those who do decide to stay in this undefined area it can sometimes get complicated (as we'll explore in further detail in chapter 7), and questions can arise as to whether it would be best to keep things in a friendship space or return to a romantic relationship.

If you're thinking about opening that door up again with your ex-partner, then here are some questions to ask yourself:

- **'Have we both grown?'** – Are you both emotionally ready to close the door on the version of the relationship that you shared before and start a new chapter? This involves communication, talking through what went wrong and where your hopes lie for the future, and making a commitment to listen to each other's needs and share the journey together going forward.

- **'Have I explored other connections?'** – Often after a break-up we seek out the comfort that the other person offered us and struggle to move on. Have you given yourself the opportunity to seek out new connections before returning to your ex? This isn't to say that you need to have gone on a certain number of dates or slept with other people to find the answer, but have you allowed yourself to open up to new possibilities and are you sure that you still feel the pull of your ex-partner? This is an important question to ask yourself, and in turn, the other person too.
- **'Do we have aligned goals for the future?'** – There's no point walking back into a relationship and beginning to date someone again if the reason it didn't work out was based on some of your core values and goals being misaligned. It's important to understand the reason for the break-up, mutually take accountability and discuss where you'd like things to head in the future by being brutally honest. Romanticising closeness and comfort is common, so you need to ground your feelings in reality to find the answers that you need as to whether your connection still has legs in the real world.
- **'Did they block me?'** – The opposite of love is not hate, it's indifference, so in the initial period after your break-up if your ex has blocked you on messaging platforms or social media, it's likely because they're trying to avoid you entirely, or because they *still have feelings*.

Reaching out to someone in the months after a break-up is tempting but you need to allow your feelings to settle and allow the other person to do some healing and growing too.

If, when you reach out, your ex is keen to meet up or still has a strong emotional reaction it's highly likely that the feelings are still there, but if you receive an indifferent response or feel that the tone between you has shifted to be somewhat nonchalant and casually indifferent, it's likely that they have started to shift how they see you and have moved on from the situation.

Either way, if you want to re-establish contact with someone then it's important to do so in a considerate and kind manner.

- **'When should I start dating again?'** – I get a lot of messages from people in my DMs asking when the appropriate time is to start dating someone again after a connection has ended, but sadly I don't have the answer. This isn't because I'm being rude, but because it really only lies with *you*.

  Social media is a wonderful tool to help us navigate our feelings but I think we've forgotten to tap into the most powerful tool we have at our disposal, and that's intuition. If you can't get someone off your mind, then you should probably tell them, and if you have been walking around like an easy breezy flower with nothing in your head for months and you meet someone who seems fun and attractive, then it's probably OK to move on from your past and see if they want to grab a drink.

  Life really is simple when you strip it back to basics and remove the noise.

Final thoughts at the end of our little date (aka this chapter)

Dating as a newly out or questioning queer woman can definitely feel intimidating and overwhelming at times. But hopefully all the advice shared here has helped make it feel a bit more manageable and less anxiety-provoking.

Remember, don't be afraid to show your true self and let people see that you care.

When you lead with honesty, kindness and genuine warmth, the right people will naturally be drawn to you.

Put yourself out there, even if it means stepping outside your comfort zone. You never know what unexpected connections and beautiful experiences might come your way when you take that leap.

Embrace the journey: you might just surprise yourself with how fun it can be!

Good luck! x

FIVE

Sex

The first time I slept with another woman I tried a bit of everything all at once. A sort of sexual buffet if you will. I'd read that you could do so much more than with a man. However, much like going to the gym for the first time, I raced around doing circuits, spent five minutes on each activity, then collapsed with cramps.

I learned very quickly that it was less about *what* you do and more about *how* you do it.

These days I'd like to think I'm pretty good in bed (I haven't received a bad review yet, unless the people I've been sleeping with are just very polite) but getting there has *definitely* been a journey of trial, error, awkwardness, hilarity but eventually confidence.

And this is exactly why I wanted to include a chapter on sex.

Even though we live in a world that's saturated with sexual content, so much of it is still vague, inaccurate or just plain unhelpful, especially if you're a queer woman, or *anyone* new to sleeping with women.

Let's be honest, mainstream references to queer sex between women are still pretty dire. It's either some over-the-top, porn-style scissoring scene or a token threesome where the man somehow ends up being the main event (which, spoiler, he never is).

Sex between two women is so often misrepresented, misunderstood or completely ignored in the conversations we grow up with, which is not just frustrating, but *exhausting*. You end up having to do all the work yourself – googling, guessing, piecing things together – all while navigating your own feelings and figuring out what actually feels good, safe and affirming. And because queer sex isn't always talked about openly, it can feel incredibly vulnerable, especially the first few times. You're not just undressing physically, you're revealing yourself emotionally too, and that can feel terrifying, thrilling and anxiety-inducing all at once.

I know from my own experience and from the many messages I get online that lots of people have questions that they're too scared to ask about sex with another woman, so that's exactly why this chapter exists: so you don't have to figure it all out on your own.

We'll cover the practical stuff, the emotional side, the awkward bits, what to do afterwards (because that's important too) and of course, ways to make good sex, *great*. Holding space for those questions, the ones you want to ask out loud but maybe don't know how to word.

Think of it as a queer sex guide written by your big sister, who's been there, made the mistakes, figured out what's fun and wants to pass on the wisdom about:

- The history of sex
- Why we struggle with the idea of sex between two women, including the role of sex ed in schools
- How to kiss another woman
- What to do before you have sex with a woman, including getting to know yourself first, learning to manage your expectations and preparing yourself physically and emotionally
- How to have sex with a woman – covering all the bases, from fingering to going down on someone, as well as having sex in specific situations, ranging from sex during your period to BDSM and threesomes
- What to do after you've had sex. From practical aftercare to addressing some questions you may now have about yourself

It's the full lowdown, without judgement, shame or assumption.

A quick history of sex (I promise it's interesting or I wouldn't have bothered writing it)

Let's start with the basics. When I looked up the phrase 'sexual intercourse' on various online dictionaries and search engines, aside from getting a recommended shortlist of adult websites to browse I found that the definition was different for each. Some claimed that sex only counted if a 'penis was inserted into a vagina', some used language like 'traditional' to describe sex between a man and a woman and some said it also constituted intercourse if you received a 'penis in your mouth'.

I truly am enlightened.

The words we use to describe sex have an interesting history that is still relevant today. According to the *Oxford English Dictionary* the word 'sex' originated around the year 1200 and at the time it simply referred to genitalia. Then came the idea of 'fornication', which in the 1300s became a prevalent phrase to describe sexual encounters between those who were not married (referring to the Latin word *fornix*, which means 'arch' – which all the prostitutes in ancient Rome allegedly liked to hang out underneath).

The word 'f*ck' wasn't found in a dictionary until 1598. Its use had Old Germanic roots with the words *ficken* or *fucken*, meaning to 'strike' or 'penetrate', further binding the language around the act of sex itself with the idea that pleasure equals force (a narrative that is still very much prevalent in society today).

We also have the Bible, the Church and religious institutions, who since conception have restricted, preached and policed access to sex, instilling the belief that lust and desire are sinful, punishable and should only occur within a tight framework of boundaries (usually set by the institution themselves to protect their power and monetary value).

They believed a woman could lie with a man, but only if you're married, prioritise his orgasm over yours, promise never to cheat (even though you're probably miserable), bear 15 children and stay quiet in the process.

Now, I'm not saying modern-day heterosexual marriages are at all like this (and if yours is then *please leave him*) but it's worth noticing how these outdated beliefs have shaped what we've been taught to view as 'normal' when it comes to sex, pleasure and desire. These ideas didn't just disappear, they seeped into our sex education, our media, our family dynamics and the way we speak (or don't speak) about queer sex today.

And maybe that's already had an effect on *you*, whether you realise it or not.

Why we struggle with the idea of sex between two women

We struggle to comprehend things that don't feel normal to us. Maybe that's why you've felt unsure about what *counts* as sex between two women. Maybe that's why no one ever explained it properly, and why you've had to do your own late-night googling or quietly gather tips from friends. Maybe that's why sex with another woman feels exciting but also a bit terrifying, not because you're doing anything wrong, but because you've absorbed the idea (like so many of us have) that anything outside the straight, penis-in-vagina norm is somehow 'less than', confusing or even invisible.

Historically, sex between women wasn't considered 'real', because it didn't lead to babies. And if something doesn't result in a family tree or a census box, then apparently it didn't count.

That lack of recognition has ripple effects: if it's not validated by society, it doesn't get talked about, taught or celebrated. It gets buried. Or turned into something for someone else's fantasy.

And this is exactly why this chapter is important.

Because if you've ever felt confused, embarrassed or even a little ashamed for not knowing what queer sex is 'supposed' to look like, I want you to know that none of that is your fault. You were never given the tools. You were never offered the language. And chances are, you've been quietly stitching together your own understanding in the dark. Guessing, googling and hoping you're doing it 'right'.

But queer sex isn't something to get right. It's something to *feel*, explore, enjoy, communicate and define in a way that feels good for you *and* your partner.

Sex education in schools

When I grew up there was very limited sex education for those who identified as LGBTQ+. I went to school in Scotland (where I was living at the time) in the 1990s under Section 28 (a law that prohibited local authorities from promoting homosexuality, including teaching its acceptability as a family relationship) and therefore I didn't have the opportunity to learn what an alternative to being with a boy looked like, because in my world it simply didn't exist: it was erased.

It was only when Section 28 was abolished in 2000 for Scotland and 2003 for England that different narratives slowly started to creep in, but even then the teaching was still focused on how to put a condom on a banana and controlling a classroom full of hysterical teenagers who were aghast at photos of sexual diseases, putting us off going within a mile of each other with a bargepole.

In 2020, Relationships and Sex Education (RSE) was made compulsory for all secondary school pupils in England, and Health Education compulsory for all pupils in state-funded schools across the country, but it is still an incredibly grey area.

Parents can also choose to withdraw their child from the teaching (for example, around gender reassignment, transgender topics and queer relationships) and the quality of the information imparted is still very much dependent on the individual leading the class and to how in-depth they decide these discussions should go.

In the USA, the landscape is more complex and ever-changing: some states mandate comprehensive sex education, including information on contraception and STIs, while others prioritise abstinence or restrict certain topics. Many states also require schools to involve parents in sex education decisions, either through consent or opt-out policies.

Regardless of where you grow up in the world, one thing is certain: many members of the LGBTQ+ community, particularly women, leave the education system none the wiser as to how to go about sex and intimacy and have the hefty task ahead of them to educate themselves through books, podcasts and social media before any real-life action actually takes place.

A lot of queer women learn what to do in the bedroom through a whole host of channels, varying from TikTok and porn sites to conversations with friends or literally learning as they go.

I for one had no idea how to be with a woman until I found out about the online magazine *Bustle,* which a friend of mine was writing for at the time and recommended I study, but even then my understanding of how sex worked was poor and I relied heavily on the openness in the community around sharing stories, tips and, funnily enough, links to spicy videos (which as a newly out queer woman, blew my mind) to send me on my way to serve up my infamous sexual buffet.

Thankfully, *this* book is now adding to the discourse, though of course all of those other means are very much valid.

A note on intimacy

When we talk about intimacy, we automatically think of sex, but physical connection only constitutes a part of the word. There are many ways to be intimate with another person without engaging in intercourse, such as kissing, hugging, holding hands and more. There are also many ways you can be intimate with another person that don't feature physicality at all, such as shared experiences, intellectual conversations or laughter. Asexuals, for example, still experience intimacy – they just prefer this intimacy to be non-sexual.

Whichever way you choose to share a connection with someone is valid and shouldn't need to depend solely on being physical. For the purpose of this chapter, though, I am going to focus on physical intimacy, and more specifically sexual connection.

MY STORY

When I was 10 I had my first kiss with a boy called Tom*. It was after Youth Club and his breath tasted like raspberry yoghurt. I was never worried about having my first 'proper' kiss because I always secretly suspected that I'd be quite good at it. Which I was. But then I realised I liked women, and the electric confidence *dulled* slightly.

Before I came out at the age of 21 I had only 'properly' kissed men. In high school I made out with the boys who everyone drooled over, yet I found it all quite boring and monotonous. My attitude was extremely nonchalant. They could have the chance to make out with me if they were lucky, but I wasn't fussed either way. I adopted a lukewarm demeanour as a deterrent, but instead of driving them away as intended, it seemed to drive them *wild* instead.

My first *proper* kiss with a girl, though, altered my brain chemistry entirely. It was heavy, hot and over a decade on, I still struggle to describe how great it was.

The year was 2015 and I'd just moved down to London. I was 21 and swiping on the dating apps with the option exclusively set to 'women' and to my surprise a tall girl with long brunette hair matched with me, and we planned a date.

Jen* had kissed women before and that intimidated me, because I wasn't really sure how to start. I'd seen on films that girls ran their fingers through each other's hair so I thought I'd give that a go. The last thing I wanted to do was stand there like a motionless HB pencil. I started; she followed.

I remember how soft her lips felt on mine, which sounds like a complete cliché, but until you make out with another woman (which I highly recommend you do), you really don't realise how different it feels. Everything about it felt amazing. Her hands were in my hair, then around my waist and unzipping my jeans.

For a long time I believed that kiss felt so incredible simply because it was with the 'right' gender. But as I've explored my sexuality more, I've come to realise that true intimacy isn't about gender, it's about the connection you share with that specific person (or people) in that moment – the elusive, electric 'spark'.

It's a spark many of us have felt when kissing a woman for the first time. I asked my community of queer women to weigh in on that moment:

QUEER VOICES

'My first kiss with another girl was in the dark back seat of a friend's car when I was in high school. Being kissed by boys always felt like they were taking something from me. Kissing her felt like we were sharing something, like a delicious little secret just for us. We held hands for ages first, caressing each other's fingers. The kiss seemed to take forever to happen and I could feel her smiling through it.'

'We were 15, best friends for five years, out to each other but terrified of the backlash if we were to be together. I had teased her the night before over text that this cute girl had kissed me. She was silent all night and for the first half hour of school the next morning. Then as we were walking to class, she grabbed my hand, pulled me into an empty music room, smacked her books down on the piano, grabbed my face and kissed me. No boy could ever make me feel the way that felt.'

No boy could ever make me feel the way that felt.

'My first real kiss with a woman that was actually romantic rather than sexual was at the end of our first date. It was like being a teenager again! Soft, slow, it took every fibre of my being to not invite her in. The second date was the next day. That ended at her house. Hot.'

'My first kiss with a girl was when I was still in the closet, but when I kissed my first girlfriend, which led me to realise I'm a lesbian, it felt like I was young again and all I wanted to do was kiss her endlessly. She had a lip ring, and one night we kissed so much it slipped out! We spent the rest of the night trying to push it back in!'

'I was 16, in a truck with my two best friends and three guys, riding along the winding country back roads. I was sitting in the lap of a guy

I'd just met that night in the front passenger seat, while my friends and one of the other guys were in the back. Two of the guys wanted to start a game of "who's the best kisser". At first it was the girls kissing the guys and then the guy I was sitting with suggested that my friend and I kiss to see who was better. We were both up for it – she was by far the better kisser, but I was way too embarrassed to admit it at the time!'

'Small-town goth night – so, slim pickings. Then she walks in: New Rock boots, leather pants, purple bra under fishnet. We locked eyes all night and finally kissed to "I Wanna F*ck You Like an Animal". And girl, honestly . . . It felt exactly like that.'

How to kiss someone and make it memorable

Obviously there are lots of ways to kiss someone, and you'll find your own preferred way, but here are some tips to get you started:

- **Rhythm** – Don't forget the power of slow breathing, rhythm and pace. Kissing doesn't have to be fast; it can actually be really hot to take it slow. Try breathing in and out together, switching up the pace or even calling out the rhythm. A favourite line of mine to drop is 'Remember to breathe', it's playful, assertive and funnily enough, always manages to elicit the exact opposite effect.
- **Eye contact** – Whether you choose to close your eyes or sporadically open them is up to you. I would, however, say that it *definitely* changes the mood if you keep them open. Your brain can focus on other sensations more when it shuts off a sense, so it's likely going to be a more pleasurable experience if you don't stare.
- **Biting** – Please be careful with lip biting. It's sexy in small doses but if you're constantly nibbling on someone's lips or ears or other areas [cough] then it's going to get a bit tiring, and painful for them. Keep it light and use it sparingly.
- **Hands in the hair** – Get your damn hands out of your pockets and run them lightly through their hair. It doesn't matter whether they have lots of it or just a bit, most people love this, but remember it's a personal thing and it might not always be appropriate or enjoyable for the other person.

> **Right person, wrong lips?**
>
> I was 26 years old when I figured out that there was such a thing as a *top* and a *bottom lip kisser*. I was kissing a girl and it suddenly didn't work. We were both top-lip women and battling to kiss. It was remarkable. I had to succumb to the bottom lip, which actually (much like that short-lived relationship) didn't really work out for me. Sometimes it doesn't flow, and that's OK.
>
> You might also see this showing up when you hold hands, with who is the 'forward' hand and who is the 'back' (although it's probably easier to navigate this than lips!).

Before you have sex with a woman

The quality of the advice that you read or watch online can be varied, so I'm here to set the record straight, based on my own experience and information I've gathered from lots of other queer women. But before we dive into the *Queerma Sutra* (see what I did there) I want to preface all of this with the following:

- Intimacy without consent is not intimacy. You need to communicate with the person (or people) you're physically connecting to, to make sure that you are all on the same page. Asking for consent is actually hot and can be part of your sexual script (as we'll go on to discuss).
- Physical intimacy can look like a one-on-one experience or it can involve more people; you make your own rules, baby.
- Intimacy thrives on mutual trust and respect (even if she's screaming 'choke me') – remember that.

Sex between two women still remains quite a mystery, not only for those who want to do it but for those who are just curious about how it works in general.

I remember a conversation in which a work colleague asked if I always keep a dildo in my backpack 'just in case' and I reacted with a howl, until I realised that she was deadly serious and had no clue how it all 'pieced together'.

So here I am, about to blow your mind with how hot your sex life can look (and no, you don't need to carry around a six-incher in your cross-body).

Get to know yourself

If you want to have good sex with another woman then you need to get to know yourself. Great sex is about being in sync with someone physically *and* emotionally, and that involves communication. You can't direct someone on what you need or know what another person might need if you have no clue what *you* like first.

Putting it simply, it's time to discover your own body and what gets you off.

Nobody ever said, 'Oh no, it's so awful having to have multiple orgasms', so it's time to set yourself some homework ...

Vibrators

According to a 2023 study by bedbible.com, 69 per cent of women in the US aged 18 to 60 have a vibrator and LGBT-identifying individuals in the USA spend 13.4 per cent more on sex products each year compared to straight people, so it's not surprising that sex toys are where I'm going to start this guide.

Vibrators come in all shapes and sizes and all achieve different results, so they can be a great way of exploring what works for you. Some people might love vibrators and others may not; at the end of the day it's all down to personal preference. At one point last year you'd have thought that I had a severe addiction to sex toys, as I had about 30 in my wardrobe because of an ongoing brand deal. (Needless to say, nearly every one of my friends, including their partners, siblings and mothers have all happily received a nice vibrator off the back of that, so using them can't be that bad.)

If you want to explore this world then I'd really recommend buying from an established brand or shop and not going cheap. This is mainly due to the quality of the materials used (i.e. the silicone and plastic).

After all, you're using these toys on and sometimes *inside* your body, so you want to make sure they're safe.

There are plenty of ethical stores out there as well as LGBTQ+- and women-owned ones, so I recommend doing your research before buying. Many of them also ship in discreet packaging, which is an obvious bonus, as nobody wants 'giant rabbit vibrator' in capital letters arriving on their front doorstep.

You can also check out sex educators on Instagram and TikTok to see what they recommend, it's also good to read the reviews for how loud they're going to be. It's probably best not to wake up your household if you're experimenting – it might be a bit of a 'buzz' kill. Pun intended.

Porn

Reading Pornhub's 2024 'Year In Review' report, the findings for what women enjoy watching globally do not come as a surprise.

The number one category viewed by women is 'lesbian'. The search term 'scissoring' was viewed a staggering 143 per cent more by female than male visitors to the site and the traffic of women to the site has seen a 2 per cent increase from 2023, making the overall split of users on the site 62 per cent male and 38 per cent female. Basically, women are watching other women with women and getting off, yet nobody is talking about it.

The topic of porn can be divisive: some people like to watch it, others don't, and for many years there have been lengthy conversations around the ethics of it. I even created a video myself talking about the way women are engaging with porn online, which incited a lot of opinions (interestingly, mainly from disgruntled men).

There should be no shame around consuming content to understand yourself better, so long as it is legal and (in my personal opinion) ethical. There are many issues in the mainstream porn space around pay, safety and the pushing of misogynistic narratives, to name a few, so it's important to recognise this.

If you are still curious, then I would encourage you to check out alternatives to the mainstream free sites.

The desire to watch porn isn't going to go away but we can do something about how we consume it in a more 'fair trade' way.

Alternatively, if you're looking for video content that is more educational and less narrative-led, then you could try apps which offer step-by-step videos and audio content to help you learn more about yourself and others.

Prepare yourself mentally

Are you ready to sleep with a woman, not just physically, but emotionally too? It's completely normal for questions to come up, especially if it's your first time. You might feel excited, nervous, unsure or all of the above. Take a moment to check in with yourself. Is this something you really want right now? If there are emotional blockers, fear, shame, confusion or performance anxiety, it's OK to pause and reflect or even talk it through with your partner if you feel safe doing so. There's no deadline or pressure, and you don't owe anyone intimacy before you're ready.

If you decide to explore that connection, know that it's completely normal for unexpected feelings to come up in the moment. Being with another woman can feel deeply validating and intimate, but also vulnerable, especially if it's new territory.

Move forwards with openness, honesty and self-compassion. Trust, respect, communication and consent are your foundation. There's no 'right' way to do it – only what feels good, safe and authentic to you both.

Health factors that can affect sex

Your mental health plays a huge role in how open, relaxed and present you can be in sexual moments, and checking in with your mindset before getting physical is crucial.

It's not just about nerves or excitement: factors like anxiety, depression or past stress can significantly dampen desire or intimacy. In fact, in the UK, almost 47 per cent of adults say health issues, including mental health, have affected their sex lives. Similarly, in the USA, up to one-third of adult women experience hypoactive sexual desire disorder (HSDD), where low desire causes distress, often linked to psychological or emotional factors.

Manage your expectations

The first time I had sex with another woman was perhaps not the experience I had pictured. Carrie* and I had been seeing each other for a few weeks. She was a petite redhead with sparkly eyes who I thought was really beautiful, so I took her out for a date to a bowling alley followed by a Turkish restaurant.

Later in the evening, we made out in our underwear to one of my homemade Spotify playlists (which was definitely the wrong tempo to have sex to). This involved some awkward moments when she nearly fell off the bed, as well as me shifting up a gear to try something new every few minutes. Then, suddenly, I started to feel *very* hot – and not in a good way.

In a state of panic, I rushed to the bathroom and violently threw up. It's a scene that will haunt me forever.

As you can see, sometimes your first sexual encounter with a woman can be clumsy, messy, hilarious and hot all at the same time. So try not to put too much pressure on yourself or your partner: go in with an open mind and have fun! I'm not alone in not having had the 'perfect' first time – as the stories from other queer women below reveal, these moments vary a lot:

QUEER VOICES

'My first time was not that great, I actually thought, I'm not lesbian at all and just admire women from afar. The reality is that we just weren't very compatible in the bedroom. When I did find someone for the second time, it was a much better experience. I was clear that I was just exploring and her response was, "Are you sure you're not a lesbian?"'

'I didn't know what I was doing, but neither did she and we were willing to laugh at ourselves the whole time. It was so much fun. We taught each other how to touch each other. It was innocent and sweet, and unlike with a guy, it was equal.'

'My first time having sex with a woman was a foursome with our boyfriends there. Somehow multi-person sex is much more acceptable when you're closeted, even though many people don't get started that way. I always negotiated with myself: I really want to be with a woman, so I need to bring a woman into my relationship with my boyfriend in order to make this happen.'

'I finally knew what it felt to be really turned on. When I was with men, it felt performative and I always hoped it would be over quickly (not surprisingly, it usually was!). After the first time with a woman, I knew that was what sex was meant to feel like.'

> **It was innocent and sweet, and unlike with a guy, it was equal.**

'It felt gentle and safe, but also far more vulnerable than I expected. Afterwards I felt weird, almost shaken, because it was pivotal.'

'It was so connected in a way I didn't realise I was missing before, when I was having sex with men. My whole body and mind were so present in the moment with her that made me enjoy the experience so much more. Every touch and every kiss felt electric, like my whole body was engulfed in desire. It made me realise that all those songs about love and sex weren't exaggerating, like I thought they were before!'

Prepare yourself physically

As discussed, it's all about setting yourself up to feel good – emotionally, mentally and physically. When you understand your own pace, what helps you feel safe and what turns you on, you're far more likely to have a positive experience (or at the very least, a funny story).

Once you've done that inner check-in, there are also a few very real, practical things you can do to make the whole situation a lot more comfortable for both of you.

Here's my sexy checklist – 'a sex-list', if you will (humour me with these titles):

- **Get your lighting down** – Do NOT, I repeat *do not*, turn the big light on. You want candles, mood lighting and small lamps. Think seductive, not hardware store lighting aisle.
- **Cut your nails** – Or at least cut the two nails that you might *[ahem]* need to use. That shit gets jabby and pointy and nobody needs that.

- **Get a hair tie on hand and place it close by** – If either of you has hair longer than shoulder length, you might need to use it to tie your hair up. Two women having sex gets hot and hair goes *everywhere*.
- **Get a good playlist cued** – And more importantly, know that the vibe works for *you*. There is nothing worse than a rogue song or wrong tempo if you're hooking up. Moody, low, deep beats are a great crowd-pleaser.
- **Hydration** – I actually sound like your mother, but seriously, stay hydrated.
- **Don't get too drunk** – Being a bit tipsy is fun and can take the edge off, but being drunk makes you sloppy and messy and clumsy and none of that is sexy. Know your limits in advance and stick with them if you want your night (or day) to be memorable for the right reasons.
- **Remember, it's a privilege for someone to have access to your body** – Own that and make sure it's respected too.
- **Have FUN** – Sometimes sex can look like someone throwing you/you throwing them against a wall and having a hot five minutes of fun. Sometimes all the rules go out of the window, so try to just roll with it!

A note on sexual health

It's a myth that women who have sex with other women shouldn't be concerned about STIs and STDs. I'm not here to scare you (in fact quite the opposite), but to tell you that you should regularly test yourself if you're sleeping with new people.

Even though the risk of transferring something through non-penetrative contact is lower with women, you are still exchanging bodily fluids and (in some cases) these could include blood if one or both of you is menstruating.

If you're in an open relationship then it's even more important for everyone involved to stay on top of their sexual health (especially if you identify as bisexual or are sleeping with multiple genders, as the types of STIs and STDs can sometimes look different).

I didn't find out that I needed to do STD tests until I met someone I worked with who enlightened me at the age of 25. Then I panicked, ordered a test online, got drunk and hurt myself by not reading the instructions properly (so don't do that).

A lot of the time these kits are available online and will be sent free of charge to your home address anonymously (in London, the local one is called SHL). You'll fill in a questionnaire and then be sent the right tests (usually a self-administered blood test and a swab) to correspond with that. It's easy, it doesn't take long and it allows you peace of mind afterwards.

If you're based in the UK, you can also go to a walk-in centre and get a test done there and then, through the NHS, charities or dedicated sexual health clinics. If you are outside of the UK then a simple google should give you the information you need to find out where to get tested.

None of this is designed to hinder your experience; it should only enhance it.

Now for the fun part – having sex with a woman

We've talked about how to prepare emotionally and physically but now you might be wondering: *What do we actually do? How does it work?* If you've never had sex with a woman before, or you've only ever seen it portrayed through unrealistic porn or vague references in pop culture, it's totally normal to feel unsure or curious. That's why this next section is here: to walk you through the practical stuff, techniques, touch, connection and everything in between.

This isn't a 'how-to' manual with rigid steps or a universal formula (because spoiler: there isn't one). But it *is* a guide to help you understand what's possible, what tends to feel good, and how to explore with confidence, respect and playfulness. It's based on my own and other queer women's experiences, which are wide-ranging and enlightening in equal measure. Let's get into it.

Fingering

Unfortunately, a lot of people out there haven't yet mastered the art of fingering and think that showing a woman a good time involves repeatedly going in and out at the same angle until something happens, or more likely, your arm becomes sore and you have to stop for fear of developing a repetitive strain injury.

Let me help...

Rose theory

Start from the outside in. There are places to visit before you go straight there, if you get my drift. Use your hands to explore all the other layers of the rose in a light-touch, no-force way. Start from the outside in and work up to what you're going to do with a bit of mystery.

Do not immediately jab.

Hand placement

Where you are lying with your partner affects how much movement your wrist has. For example, if you're lying side by side that's great because you can see their face and understand if what you're doing is working, but your wrist is going to get sore pretty soon. You might want to experiment with being a little lower down to give your wrist more flexibility, sitting or even standing.

These little things actually make a big difference.

The 'come here' movement

I'm not suggesting you hook your partner like your hand is a claw, but you do want to do a slight 'come here' motion with your finger rather than just going in and out and hurting them. The 'come here' motion is essentially a stroke that stimulates the G spot.

Give it a go. I promise, your partner will thank you.

Licking your fingers

That surprised you, didn't it?

[This is the point where I'm acutely aware of a conversation I had with my mother, in which she mentioned that her friends at the local crafting club couldn't wait to read this book.]

Should you lick your fingers when you're fingering another woman?

Some of you might be screwing your face up and others nodding in agreement at the idea. It's a preference you need to figure out with your partner.

There's no guide on how to do this but I wanted to include it here to dissipate any awkwardness or shame that might linger.

Some people find it really hot and some not so much. I guess you'll never know until you try...

Scissoring and tribbing

We've all heard the jokes around pairs of scissors and lesbians but let's unpack what it actually means... and more importantly, how you actually do it.

First, this isn't an activity exclusive to lesbians; it's available to *anyone* who wants to grind down there in an 'interlocked way' and explore.

Scissoring refers to direct contact between your vulva and the other person's vulva (I'm aware this sounds like a science lesson now but there really isn't any way around it) and it's usually done with one person lying down and the other quite literally sliding their legs in between and grinding on top.

There are a few things to note with scissoring, though. The first is that it does take a certain amount of co-ordination, which if you're new to the scissor game is going to need some banter and a good sense of humour to navigate because it might take some time to 'line up' with the other person.

It also takes some stamina to continually maintain contact and the person on top usually ends up doing most of the work, but what *can* sometimes help (if you're a little inflexible) is to place a vibrator between you both when you're in the middle of it.

Tribbing, on the other hand, is probably more likely what will happen. It refers to a sort of grinding on each other's thighs, hips or other similar bodily areas. It's sometimes easier but it really is a case of figuring out how you 'flow' with your partner; everyone is different.

As you're probably starting to realise, there isn't one 'specific' way to be physically intimate with a person (or people), and thankfully there are plenty of options available to you!

Going down

This is the big one (even though it doesn't really need to be), and it's often one of the main reasons that newly out women fear being intimate with another woman, as the pressure to be able to do this seems intense.

Thankfully, I'm no stranger to this topic, as one of my most viral videos on TikTok (amassing over 13 million views) directly talks about how to do this well, so you're in safe hands as we unpack it.

First, you *do not* have to do anything that you're not into, nor do you have to give or be on the receiving end of this one activity in order to validate your sexual identity. It's simply part of the wider offering of how women can have sex with each other, and like the other things I've covered, it's there for you to pick up *if* and *when* you feel comfortable.

How to start

Start with some kissing. Go from her neck down the body and linger a bit around her lower abdomen. Maybe you can flash a little smile at this point – keep her interested. You don't want to go straight in, so build up a bit of tension.

Rhythm and pace

There is too much advice out there about how you need to spell out the alphabet with your tongue, go between wide licking and more 'pointed' licking or stop halfway through to twirl around and come back to it. It's f*cking overwhelming, so let's simplify it.

Start slowly and build your way up. I'm no sexpert (she says, having written a chapter on it) but it's probably worth switching between having a slow flat tongue and a slightly pacier lick. Either way you can probably gather the reaction from your partner by the visuals and noises that they're making, so I'd lead with that, rather than a choreographed routine.

Helping hand

Sometimes it can be a physically hard task to help someone reach orgasm using only your tongue. Think about it: it's a lot. This is why there should be no shame about doing a hybrid of hand action and mouth action. Women do it with men, so what's the problem here? Sometimes it feels good to mix things up in the moment too, especially if it's been a hot minute.

Eye contact

This leads me next to eye contact. This can be *super-hot* in small doses throughout, but dear lord, do not give prolonged wide-eye contact like you've witnessed a crime, because it sure as hell will put the other person off.

Go with the vibe and close your eyes; enjoy yourself too.

Pillow trick

It's nice to be nice. Sometimes it helps if you place a pillow under your partner's lower back. It just offers a bit more support and also makes the angle a bit easier.

One awkward question

Yep, I knew it was coming. 'What if it smells bad, or I smell bad, or the whole world collapses and I go into meltdown?' This is definitely a possibility (as it is when you're intimate with anybody) but it's highly unlikely that your natural odour is going to put your partner off or, if I'm honest, they will even notice it.

If you want to feel great about yourself then freshen up before you sleep together, but it's not the end of the world if you don't. Sometimes things happen in the moment and you can't always be perfect and prepared.

If they comment negatively on this or use it as an excuse not to sleep with you again then you definitely don't want to be with them anyway.

Do you need a dick?

If you want one, then yes, but also, you don't have to either.

Buying a dildo can sometimes be embarrassing or difficult. It shouldn't be, but there's still a stigma around it. This stems mainly from the idea that the reproduction of the male organ is an abomination, and that dildos completely serve women and will only encourage indecent behaviour. Although I'd disagree that reproducing dicks (even though a dildo technically isn't a dick – it's just shaped the same) is an abomination, I can get behind the other two reasons: they're probably why you *should* buy a dildo in the first place.

Let me be real with you. Dildos (like dicks) come in varying qualities. The more you spend, the better the quality will be, and also (as I mentioned in the section about vibrators on p. 143) the better the quality of the materials too.

If you do decide to go down the purchasing route then there are a couple of things to consider. Number one, the size. Toys are made for people of all shapes and builds (it's not a one-size-fits-all situation), so make sure you go for something that feels comfortable. This isn't a competition; you don't have to buy the biggest dildo in the shop to prove that you're more 'sexually liberated'. Just get something that feels right and not overwhelming!

Second, you'll want to get some lubrication that doesn't break down silicone (the material that most of these toys are made out of).

Third, you'll need a way of wearing it. There are usually two options. The first is a harness that you can tighten with straps, although it can be quite tricky for beginners and I wouldn't recommend it as it involves a lot of buckles or Velcro (and might lead to the other person having a tea break and popping to the bathroom in the time that you get it on) and the second option (and the one I'd recommend for first-timers) is a pair of boxer shorts that have a hole and hold it in place for you.

Usually if you purchase something online then it will pop up with a recommended way of wearing it, but if not, just check the details and match it to the right pair of boxers. Also, downsize your boxers a bit, because if they're too big and slip off then the whole thing will be a shitshow. Granted it will be hilarious, but definitely not hot.

Specific scenarios

All of the above are pretty common techniques that are spoken about in the community, but what about specific situations that perhaps get less airtime? Let's take a look at a few now:

Period sex

Having sex on your period can actually be a really intimate and erotic experience, yet for many of us, we tend to mark it as, quite literally, a 'period' of the month when sex is off the cards. Social stigma, discomfort or just plain habit often lead people to avoid it altogether. But with a little planning (such as covering the sheets or using a dark towel), period sex can not only be enjoyable, but it also carries some surprising benefits, both physically and emotionally.

For one, orgasms during menstruation can help relieve cramps. This happens because orgasm involves uterine muscle contractions, which promote the release of built-up menstrual blood and increase blood flow to the uterus, both of which can reduce the intensity of cramps and even help shorten the duration of your period. In fact, studies have shown that orgasm releases endorphins, which act as natural painkillers and mood-boosters, helping with both physical symptoms and emotional ones, such as irritability and fatigue.

Interestingly, for some people, libido can actually spike during menstruation. This is likely due to fluctuations in oestrogen and testosterone, hormones that can increase sensitivity and arousal in the days leading up to and during your period. According to a survey by Clue (a menstrual tracking app) and the Kinsey Institute, 'around 30% of people report feeling more sexually aroused during their period', and many also report stronger orgasms due to heightened sensitivity.

So if you're feeling curious, this could be the perfect time to explore, as long as the desire is there and communication is open with your partner. As with anything sexual, comfort, consent and clear boundaries are key. Not everyone will feel comfortable with the idea of period sex, and that's completely OK – it's not for everyone. But if both partners are on board, there's no reason it should be off the table.

Of course, because blood is likely to be present (and potentially exchanged), it's important to practise safe sex, especially if you're not in a mutually monogamous relationship or haven't been tested. With a little care and openness, period sex can be another way to connect more deeply, with your body, your pleasure and your partner.

Shower sex

I feel like the art of shower sex is dying, or perhaps people don't talk about it as much as they used to, and I think that's a shame.

When I worked with a large sex toy brand a few years ago they sent me a replacement for my shower head, which not only could be used in the traditional sense to clean your body and wash yourself but also doubled up as a massager if you took it off the hook.

I personally only filmed the toy in its box and then palmed it off to a friend of mine (who sent me quite a few messages to make sure it was saved for her) and I believe it got a very good review.

It made me think that we could do a lot more in the bathroom if we tried, and although there's nothing particularly to note about this being a specific activity for two women, I do think it's hot and you should try it sometime.

'Choke me, Daddy'

There's no real distinction between practising BDSM (bondage and discipline, dominance and submission, and sadism and masochism), kink or fetish between two women versus a man and a woman. At its core, the same principles apply: mutual interest, clear communication and enthusiastic consent. Once those are in place, it's simply about exploring what feels good for both of you.

When we think of BDSM and kink, our minds might gravitate towards a landscape dominated by leather, rope or the image of a playroom as seen in *Fifty Shades of Grey*. But between two women, the scripts that play out can often be much more subtle, and that doesn't make them any less intriguing or intense. In fact, a 2021 study published in the *Journal of Homosexuality* found that around '53% of lesbian and queer women have engaged in BDSM-related activities', highlighting just how common and accepted kink is within the community.

For those new to sex with women, especially if your previous partners were men, there can be a subtle shift in the 'sexual scripts' you might expect. This doesn't need to be confusing or complicated. In fact, it's an opportunity to move away from pre-set gendered roles and instead co-create experiences based on mutual pleasure and shared curiosity.

What I find especially fascinating about power play in the queer female space is how roles like dominant and submissive often defy traditional expectations. In mainstream culture, gender expression is frequently used as a shortcut to assume sexual dynamics: masc equals dominant, femme equals submissive. But in reality, these assumptions rarely hold up. I know stereotypically 'masculine'-presenting women who love to be dominated by their partners, and 'femme fatales' who confidently call the shots in the bedroom.

Even in age-gap relationships, where one might assume the older partner holds more perceived sexual authority, it's not uncommon to see that dynamic completely flipped.

Laying my cards on the table, if you were to take a cross-section of my queer female friends and chart where they land on the kink spectrum, you'd find that many identify as 'switches'.

In other words, they're open to trying new things, flipping roles and having fun with it. And honestly? That feels like the most accurate representation of what queer women do best: we adapt, explore and embrace fluidity.

One of the most liberating parts of exploring kink as a queer woman is how open and accepting the LGBTQ+ community already is. Within these circles, honest conversations about desires, boundaries and preferences, especially when it comes to the bedroom, are not only encouraged but often celebrated. This openness makes it much harder for shame or stigma to take root.

I have friends who accompany each other to kink events and play parties purely for support, and while straight women can absolutely do this too, there's something uniquely powerful about the queer female experience. There's an unwavering sense of solidarity, the kind that says, 'I've got you, no matter what you're into this week.'

For people in heterosexual spaces, finding a sex-positive, non-judgemental community might take time. But in many queer spaces, that support system is already there – primed, ready and willing to offer lived experience and encouragement.

At the end of the day, all fantasies and sexual scripts are valid, as long as they're built on mutual consent, understanding and a shared desire to explore. Stepping into different roles, whether dominant, submissive or somewhere in between is common for women who sleep with women. And it's something that should be fun, playful and completely your own.

The most important part of all of this? Communication. What really gets you going, and what gets your partner going?

Good sex relies on good communication, before, during and after. When you keep those lines open, you're far less likely to fall into patterns that don't serve either of you. You're more likely to co-create experiences that are fulfilling, safe and exciting.

In short: kink between women isn't a different game, it's just played with different rules. Rules that are written in real time, by two (or more) people who are willing to explore, listen and evolve together.

Threesomes

Group sex takes a bit of co-ordination, and at times, choreography, to work well.

Threesomes (or more) often sound amazing in theory, but in practice, they usually take a few tries to feel natural. There's a different kind of energy in the room when more than two people are involved, and it can feel more exposing than anything you've experienced before, so it's normal for things to feel a little clunky at first while you figure out the flow.

As a queer woman, a threesome can look however you want it to. I know lesbian couples who've invited a man into the bedroom, bisexual couples who've shared an experience with another bisexual person, and single women who've played the role of the 'unicorn', usually a bisexual woman joining an existing couple, regardless of whether that couple identifies as queer or not.

My advice? Get comfortable in your sexual identity and in one-on-one sex before exploring threesomes or group dynamics. There are plenty of great resources out there if you're curious: Ruby Rare's *The Non-Monogamy Playbook*, *Polywise* by Jessica Fern or *The Ethical Slut* by Dossie Easton and Janet Hardy (which is especially useful for couples considering opening up their relationship), to name a few. But, in my opinion, the most important starting point is feeling grounded and confident in yourself.

It's also vital that everyone involved is genuinely on the same page. As a friend of mine recently said, 'It's difficult when one of them is really hot, and you just want to kick the other out of bed.' Laugh as you will, but it's a reminder of how important open communication, clear boundaries and honest intentions are when exploring these spaces.

Nobody wants to be a third wheel, especially when you're naked.

How do men fit into this?

Like many queer women, my first sexual encounter was with someone of the opposite sex, and although I won't claim it was the best sex I've ever had, it wasn't awful either.

This can sometimes feel very confusing once you've come out though, and questions can run through your mind of whether or not you *actually* enjoyed something or whether you were pre-conditioned to think you enjoyed it. If, indeed, you did enjoy it – which can be questionable with first-time sex, no matter who the partner is!

Just remember, though, just as there is a spectrum for identifying as straight, gay, bisexual, lesbian and more, there is also a spectrum for who you enjoy being physically intimate with, and sometimes the two can look very different.

I know many women who identify as lesbian but enjoy occasionally sleeping with men, gay men who regularly partake in threesomes with women, and heterosexual couples who (are arguably perhaps not as heterosexual as they think), invite both men *and* women into their dynamic.

It's OK to hold space for what you enjoy physically without it having to define your entire identity. It's also OK to recognise that sex can be a fluid experience, and physically connecting with many types of people might just mean that you're more open than you thought.

Also, just because you enjoyed something previously, it doesn't mean that you have to erase those memories or give them any more weight than what was felt in the moment.

None of the above defines who you are, nor does it erase any part of your sexuality.

After you've had sex with another woman

So, you've had sex with a woman – now what? You may now be feeling more confident, affirmed in your identity and ready for more, or you might still be feeling a little confused or unsure. Both are totally normal and common. However you feel, it's worth giving yourself a little time and care to reflect on the experience.

Sexual aftercare

Aftercare is the intentional care and attention you give to yourself and your partner(s) after any sexual experience. It means tuning in to the emotional, physical and psychological needs that arise once the act is over.

Whether sex is casual or deeply intimate, aftercare helps create a safe space for vulnerability, connection and healing. It can involve anything from cuddling, talking or quietly sharing space, to checking in emotionally or physically.

The importance of aftercare becomes especially clear when we consider the complex feelings and dynamics that sex can stir up, particularly for those exploring new aspects of their identity or navigating unfamiliar territory.

Sex is never just sex: it always carries something deeper. Sure, it can range from quick and casual to slow and emotional, but it's never as simple as two bodies moving together. There's always more beneath the surface.

The roles we take on in the bedroom are vast, as are the desires, thoughts and emotions that come with them. Our upbringing, religious background, past experiences and current environment all shape how we engage with sex and the scripts we follow.

Sex can be deeply emotional for newly out queer women or those still exploring their identity. It's not uncommon for some to experience postcoital dysphoria (feelings of sadness or tearfulness after sex) even if the experience itself was positive and meaningful.

According to a study from Queensland University of Technology, nearly half of all women experience postcoital sadness at least once in their lives, with some reporting (often inexplicable) tears during or after sex several times a month.

For queer women, this can be alarming, making you wonder if the experience was negative. However, postcoital crying can have many causes, including overwhelming emotions, hormonal shifts after orgasm or even a trauma response.

And when we say trauma, we don't necessarily mean sexual or emotional abuse. It could simply mean carrying an identity that hasn't felt authentic for many years, and the physical release of sex with another woman allowing you to process some of this for the first time.

Regardless of how you feel after sex, aftercare is an essential part of the experience, especially if you're new to sleeping with women.

Aftercare can take many forms, such as:

- Cuddling or massaging
- Taking a shower (alone or together)
- Checking in emotionally to see how you and your partner are feeling
- Sharing a non-physical activity afterwards, such as watching a movie or ordering takeout

Aftercare looks different for everyone, but practising it can foster emotional intimacy, reduce stress and improve overall sexual satisfaction – which is why it's worth making it part of your routine.

Common questions

A question that comes up time and time again for women is that if they have only had sex with a woman once, does that make them gay?

This conversation is far from new. French writer and philosopher Voltaire (who was rumoured to have had sex with an Englishman) was once asked if he'd repeat the experience. He allegedly (though this is widely contested) replied, 'Doing it once, I'm a philosopher; doing it twice, I'm a sodomite.' The implication is that enjoyment for him didn't matter – what truly revealed his identity was the choice to either leave it there or do it again.

Personally, I don't believe that the number of times you do something defines your level of desire. We're all entitled to explore and see how experiences sit with us. What truly matters isn't how often we do something, but the meaning we give it when we're honest with ourselves.

I've also had a lot of conversations with queer women who wonder if their sexual identity needs to change after a one-time hook-up with a man. Usually the uncertainty centres around the physical enjoyment they felt from the connection with the opposite sex, and the shame that follows.

It's almost as if we've chosen a sexual identity and then the very act of going against that or expanding it is as sinful and taboo as the idea of homosexuality in the first place.

My response to this is that we spend an awful lot of time and energy trying to define ourselves and understand our feelings, but how liberating would it be to just go with the flow and allow yourself to experience pleasure without judgement?

Having a relationship, dating or sleeping with women yet still having thoughts about men is totally normal regardless of your sexual orientation (and vice versa if you switch the genders around). Our minds wander through all kinds of possibilities on a daily basis – some we decide to explore, and others we simply let pass.

The brain–body disconnect

To potentially add to the confusion you may feel about having sex, what your body does and what your brain experiences during sex don't always match up. There's a term for this – non-concordance – and it's wild how common it is. According to sex educator Emily Nagoski, about 90 per cent of cis women (and 50 per cent of cis men) experience some level of mismatch between physiological arousal and subjective desire or pleasure.

Basically, just because your body is responding doesn't mean your brain is on the same page or vice versa.

That disconnect can be confusing regardless of who you're having sex with, but it can be especially confusing the first few times you're intimate with a woman. You might feel 'wet' without feeling turned on, or mentally ready but still not have a physical response.

This isn't you doing something wrong: it's biology, conditioning or just part of being human, so take reassurance in that.

SEX

Some hot thoughts to leave you with

Physical intimacy is a rich, complex and deeply personal experience. Everyone brings their own unique desires, needs, fears and hopes to the moment. Sharing that kind of closeness can feel especially vulnerable, and even more so if it's your first time being with another woman.

That said, it's important to remember the foundation that makes any intimate experience truly meaningful: consent, communication and pleasure. When these three elements are present, you can trust that the intimacy you give and receive will be a source of growth, learning and joyful exploration.

But beyond all the practicalities, don't forget to have fun – because that's often where the magic truly happens. Allow yourself to let go a little, be curious and follow where your connection takes you without overthinking it.

It's OK to laugh, to be silly and to enjoy the moment fully. Sometimes the best experiences come from loosening the reins and embracing the unknown.

So, take a deep breath, relax and enjoy the ride (pun intended). This is your journey – a chance to discover more about yourself and the beautiful, intimate connections you can create with others.

SIX

Relationships

Just when you think you've figured out the whole dating and sex thing, along comes someone who wants to take things deeper and actually define the connection.

Exciting? Yes.

Mildly terrifying? Also yes.

Starting your first queer relationship (or even second, third or fourth for that matter) can feel like a wild mix of excitement, nerves and pure thrill. It's natural to feel totally mixed up and have a collection longer than a child's Christmas list of questions that you'd like answering, but don't worry – thankfully that's where this chapter comes in! My community and I can give you the lowdown from lots of different angles and hopefully answer many of your burning questions.

The word 'relationship' can mean many different things to different people, so as you read through this chapter, I encourage you to interpret the word in whatever way feels most true for you. Every relationship is unique. Some are rooted in emotional intimacy, others in physical connection, and many exist somewhere in between. A relationship might be monogamous, polyamorous, open or something less easily defined. What matters most is not how it's labelled, but whether it's honest, authentic and safe for everyone involved.

Great relationships between two women – like most, regardless of gender – are often built on a blend of intimacy, shared values, emotional and physical connection, common goals and the ability to support one another through life's ups and downs. Letting someone into your world should feel like it adds value to your life, rather than taking away from it.

That doesn't mean every moment will be easy, but the right person will challenge you to grow, help you feel seen and encourage you to stay open, even when things get tough. And no matter whether a relationship lasts a week or a decade, it has the potential to leave a lasting imprint, shaping how we see ourselves, how we connect with others and what we come to believe we deserve in love.

If you're a queer woman navigating romantic relationships, this chapter is for you. Whether you're entering your first relationship with another woman, exploring emotional closeness in a new way or simply trying to understand what healthy queer love can look like, know that you're not alone in feeling curious or unsure.

There's no shortcut to the perfect connection. Relationships take time, effort and a willingness to learn, not just about someone else, but about yourself. Sometimes we grow through closeness, compromise and connection. Other times, it's through discomfort, discovering what we don't want and where our boundaries lie.

That's all part of the process.

You might be stepping into this space with questions, fears or a sense of nervousness that you haven't quite figured out yet. But here's the truth: you've already been building the skills for meaningful connection your whole life. Every friendship, every moment of trust, every person you've let in has taught you something about love, vulnerability and emotional intimacy.

If you're feeling uncertain, think about someone you care deeply about – someone you once didn't even know. That closeness didn't appear overnight. It grew through time, trust and shared experience.

You've done it before, and you can do it again.

So, let's start unpacking what relationships between women can really look like. We'll explore all sides of it:

- The connection and the complexity in relationships between two women and the patterns that can show up
- The green flags to look out for at the start of and during a relationship, both in yourself and the other person
- Different attachment styles – what they are, and what they mean

- Entering a long-term relationship with another woman, and the warning signs to look out for
- Questioning if the relationship is right for you, and knowing if and when to end it if it's not
- Navigating a break-up

Relationships between two women

Relationships between women have long been misunderstood or misrepresented by wider society. They're often either overly sexualised, viewed through the lens of the male gaze, or dismissed entirely, as though intimacy between two women isn't 'serious' or 'real'.

In some spaces, they're even ignored or judged more harshly than heterosexual relationships, with assumptions that they're unstable, overly emotional or less valid.

Social media plays a complicated role in shaping how these relationships are perceived. On the one hand, it has helped increase visibility, representation and community for queer women, but on the other hand, it could be argued that it has somewhat reinforced the narrative that relationships between women are dramatic, toxic or doomed from the start.

From viral memes about 'U-Haul lesbians' (lesbian couples who move in together very quickly after starting a relationship) to TikToks about taking five years to process a break-up, there's a culture of irony and dark humour around queer love, and while some of it is funny because it reflects real experiences, it also risks flattening those experiences into stereotypes.

Yes, it's true that many in the LGBTQ+ community navigate mental health challenges, often rooted in years of marginalisation, internalised shame or lack of support, and these can show up in our relationships. Some dynamics may involve unhealed trauma, attachment issues or emotional intensity that others might not fully understand.

But that's not the full story.

Because just as often, relationships between women are nurturing, supportive and safe. They're built on emotional intimacy, chosen family and shared understanding. Some couples are fiery and expressive; others are soft and steady. Like any kind of relationship, they vary widely, and no one version is more 'real' or valid than another.

What *is* universal, though, is the importance of recognising when a relationship is working, and when it's not. Just like any relationship, queer partnerships benefit from honest reflection, mutual respect and the ability to assess whether your connection is helping you grow or holding you back.

And that's exactly what we're going to unpack here: the dynamics, the challenges, and the honest reality of what it takes to build and sustain relationships between women. This matters because the intricate parts of queer relationships are so often overlooked. Either they're not given space at all, or they're romanticised as 'easier' simply because they involve two women who are assumed to automatically understand one another.

To get us started, I've included some stories of how other queer women met their partners or important people in their lives, to show that lasting same-sex attraction doesn't always start or develop in the same way:

QUEER VOICES

'I went to a party in Notting Hill about a year ago and at the end of the night outside the venue I met a beautiful woman. We started talking about life and living in London as neither of us are from here. We chatted for hours, to the point that we didn't notice that we were the last two people in the venue. So we decided that we would continue our conversation over a date – it turns out we have a lot of things in common.'

'I had recently moved to the city and wanted to try rock climbing. I didn't even know it was a gay thing. I specifically went on a night for women to climb together. I saw this really cute girl across the gym and tried not to feel nervous. Eventually, we were on the same wall and I noticed she was wearing a shirt from move-in week at

my non-local university. We had attended the same school at the same time! We got to chatting, and at the end of the night, she gave me her number. Within a month, I knew we were soulmates. Three years and way too much "will they/won't they" later, we are clearly platonic, but I couldn't be happier with that.'

'We met through an ex – not unique at all in the queer community!'

'I once briefly met a girl in a lesbian bar in NYC (I live in England, and she lived in North Carolina). We exchanged numbers and decided to meet up again in NYC for New Year's Eve. So we rented a room from Craigslist and spent a week there on our first date. We tried not to kiss until midnight because we thought a first kiss under the fireworks at midnight would be amazing, but couldn't wait. The relationship didn't last long, but it had a big impact on me!'

'I first saw Joy* at an arts festival, where she was curating spoken word, and felt drawn to her. We connected on Instagram, slowly moved from liking posts to DMs, and eventually arranged to meet at an event in my town, both assuming the other likely wanted to hang out as just friends. When I sat down across from her in the park with the tea she'd bought me, it felt like being struck by lightning – a feeling we both, unknowingly, described the same way to our friends. The connection was immediate and natural, and from that moment on there was never any question: we were all in.'

As you've probably noticed by now, relationships can begin and evolve in all kinds of ways. Throughout this chapter, I'll be weaving in moments from my own relationships with different women, because each one has offered its own lessons, tensions and points of clarity.

There have been moments in my life when relationships have had me dancing on furniture, laughing, smiling and feeling fully alive, and moments where I've found myself standing in empty apartments that no longer looked like the place I'd once called home.

I've had friends hold me while I cried uncontrollably into their laps, and I've raised a toast to the endings of relationships that stripped me of my worth, celebrating the fact that I finally walked away.

But the point of sharing these moments isn't to paint queer relationships as inherently complicated, dramatic or doomed. The point is that every connection we form has the potential to teach us, shape us and sometimes even redirect us, and that's a journey many queer women will recognise.

I know that for some readers, this may be your first time entering a relationship with a woman, and for that reason, I felt it was important to offer insights (both from my own experience and my community) that hold both light and shade. This isn't about reinforcing tired stereotypes; it's about being honest. Too often, we're shown only one side of the story: the romanticised version or the chaotic clichés. But real life unfolds in the middle. And if you ever find yourself in a difficult dynamic, I don't want you to think it's just you. These things do come up, and they don't make your relationship, or you, any less valid.

So as we move through this chapter, I'll highlight the positive things to look for in relationships, as well as the more challenging patterns and dynamics that may surface. Not as warnings, but as invitations: to notice, to reflect, and to explore how they might appear in your own life and how you can meet them with greater self-awareness, curiosity and care.

But before we explore the dynamics, challenges and joys that queer relationships can hold, let's take it back to the beginning: to the moment where something real first starts to take shape. From there, we can trace the arcs that follow the highs, the lows, and everything in between.

How to spot green flags

The early stages of a relationship between two women can be incredibly intense and exciting. There's a unique energy in those first moments of connection, the thrill of discovering another person, the rush of attraction and the feeling that something really special might be unfolding.

Psychologically, this rapid pace – often jokingly called 'U-Hauling' in queer communities –can sometimes be explained through attachment theory (see p. 178) and the human need for belonging. But it's important to emphasise that attachment theory is only one small part of a much wider picture.

The tendency for relationships to move quickly can stem from a complex blend of societal, cultural, psychological and community-specific factors. Research shows that individuals with anxious attachment styles – common in LGBTQ+ populations due to experiences of marginalisation, stigma, and the ongoing process of identity validation – may be more inclined to seek rapid intimacy to feel secure. But there are many additional layers at play.

For instance, social and cultural contexts matter. Queer women often grow up with limited models of healthy same-sex relationships, face periods of invisibility or suppression, or spend years without spaces where they can express their identity freely. When they finally find someone who sees and understands them, the urge to 'catch up' on lost time can naturally intensify the desire to move fast. Community dynamics, like the importance of chosen family, the need for emotional safety, and the scarcity of queer spaces, can also accelerate relationship milestones.

With all that intensity, it can sometimes be hard to tell what's really going on beneath the surface. Is it a genuine connection? Lust? The relief of finally feeling understood? Or something more complicated, like trauma bonding? These experiences can blur together, making it tricky to navigate your feelings clearly.

Because of this, it's helpful to pay attention to green flags – those encouraging signals that show the relationship has a healthy foundation. And on the flip side to this, what I prefer to call 'warning signs' rather than red flags, that might indicate something isn't quite right – whether at the start of the relationship or further down the line.

In this chapter, we're going to explore both, so you can better understand what to look out for as you build connections that feel good, grounded and authentic.

MY STORY

The first time I had a serious relationship with a woman, I was in my twenties. Things moved fast, and at the start it all felt refreshing and uncomplicated compared to some of the situations I'd found myself in before.

But being in a relationship with a woman for the first time was a steep learning curve. I had no idea what to expect and, in many ways, felt like a pre-pubescent teenager trying to find my footing. In the first few months, I lived on WhatsApp, constantly messaging my lesbian and bi friends for advice, trying to understand my feelings, navigate new conversations, and check whether what I was experiencing was normal.

One of my biggest challenges was figuring out whether I was truly ready for something deeper, and how to tell if someone was actually the right fit for me.

These kinds of questions often don't have straightforward answers, and even after talking them through, much of the clarity comes from listening to your own intuition and emotional signals. So before jumping in, it can be helpful to pause and turn inwards: observe how your body reacts, what thoughts arise and the kind of energy you experience when you're around them.

Green flags to look out for in yourself

When you're getting to know someone new, it's just as important to pay attention to how *you* feel in yourself as it is to observe them. Do you feel calm, grounded and like you can be fully yourself? Are you excited to share – not to impress, but to connect? Do you feel safe setting boundaries, and curious rather than anxious about where things might go?

Here are some of the healthy things I look out for in myself at the beginning of a new relationship and then we'll hear from other queer women for their take on what healthy signals look like too.

Your nervous system feels relaxed in their presence

If there is something about their presence that makes you feel safe (maybe they listen and hold space for you and you feel that your vulnerabilities aren't judged), then this is a great sign that your energies are aligned. That kind of mutual, open space is the foundation for trust and love, and it's exactly what's needed if you want the connection to grow.

Time disappears

If the chat flows so effortlessly that time just slips away, chances are it's more than just good conversation. Unless they've secretly got a TED Talk under their belt, it's likely that you probably have a lot in common. Getting lost in time is a classic sign that you're fully engaged in the connection as everything else fades into the background. (Cue memories of standing in the freezing cold or pouring rain with someone I really cared about – and barely noticing a thing!)

You're reflecting on the connection in a thoughtful, grounded way

If you're taking time to check in with your emotions and assess how open you feel to deepening the relationship, that in itself is a sign of emotional awareness: you're not just swept up in the moment or ignoring your instincts.

It's entirely healthy to ask yourself how you feel in someone else's presence, whether the connection is romantic or platonic, especially if you're uncertain or considering what the next steps might look like. (For more on this, see chapter 7.)

Your intuition and gut instincts can be powerful guides here. I've had times where I felt intensely drawn to someone, yet there was still a quiet, persistent feeling that something was off, whether it was the way they communicated or how they showed up. Learning to tune into those subtle cues is important. Often, your body picks up on things before your mind does, so don't underestimate the internal signals you already have access to.

You enjoy your own company

Not everyone enjoys being alone (though if you saw my apartment, I might just make a convincing case for it), but we *can* get comfortable with who we are, what we like and, more importantly, how we enjoy spending our time.

Starting a relationship with someone shouldn't feel like they're 'completing' you, but rather 'complementing' you. Picture them as the icing and cherry on top of the cake (and the cake is you, by the way). If you feel just as at ease on your own as you do with them, it's a strong sign that you're ready to deepen your connection, and that they respect your independence and personal journey as well.

If you feel good

This is such a simple one but we forget to ask ourselves this question: *Does this person and situation make me feel happy and good?* Of course life can't be happy and positive all of the time, but if you find yourself feeling anxious and stressed more often than you're enjoying the connection, then it's probably not the healthiest foundation to build on.

Of course, every relationship goes through periods of ups and downs, that's completely normal. But if it feels like it's *all* downs and no ups, that's a clear sign something isn't serving you. My friend and I have a simple question we use to check in on how someone makes us feel:

'Are you having fun?'

At first, that might sound a bit shallow, but what we really mean is, 'Is this person on the whole, making you, your mental health and your life better overall?' Because if the answer is no, then it's important to seriously question why you're continuing to engage with them in the first place.

'Green flags' to look out for in others

As well as checking in on your own green flags, you need to pay attention to how the other person is behaving and be on the lookout for both green flags and warning signs. Below are a few great green flags that indicate the person might make a good partner going forwards:

They communicate how they feel about you and don't leave you guessing

Now, not everyone is a great communicator and we need to take that into consideration when talking about expressing feelings and emotions. However, what we can look out for, especially in the queer dating space, is a *willingness* to grow, be vulnerable and open up. You can recognise this willingness in someone by how they *show up* for you. If they listen, hold your feelings with respect and express genuine interest in your life as well as being open (within reason, when you first start dating!) about their own experiences then these are all really great signs.

Actions to back up words

It's not words that hold the weight, but the actions that accompany them. If someone follows through on their promises, shows up when you need them and treats you with kindness and care (not just for one night, by the way – we're talking *prolonged* respect and care) then they're likely a keeper.

If their actions go against what they have shared or there is deception or lying involved, then it's not a great sign, is it?

They can talk about their ex-partner

Navigating ex-partners in the queer dating scene can feel unusual, as conventional dating 'rules' often don't apply in the same way.

While there aren't solid statistics on exactly how many queer women stay friends with their exes, several studies suggest this is a common pattern. In a study called 'LGBTQI+ break-up assemblages', many queer women described continuing emotional ties and practical relationships with ex-partners, from co-parenting pets to sharing social spaces. A more general study by Mogilski & Welling in 2017 found that people (regardless of gender or sexuality) often 'stay friends with their exes due to emotional reliability, shared history, or mutual support'. So, while exact numbers are unclear, the *trend* is very real, and it reflects the often fluid, non-traditional nature of queer relationships.

Navigating the same-sex dating scene, especially if you're new to it, can feel confusing at times. Feelings like jealousy or envy are completely normal, particularly if the person you're into still has a close bond with their ex. I wish I could say there's never anything to worry about (and often, there isn't), but as we'll explore in chapter 7, the boundaries between friendship and romance in queer female relationships can be quite fluid and from my own experience, things are often rarely straightforward or clear-cut.

One green flag to look out for is how someone speaks about their exes. This is true across the board, regardless of sexuality, because speaking openly about an ex is a strong sign of emotional maturity. But in queer spaces, where communities often overlap and relationships can evolve into friendships, this becomes even more important. The way someone talks about a past partner or close friend can tell you a lot about their values and emotional insight.

If your partner can openly reflect on their previous relationship, explain what led to its end, and clearly define where things stand now, that's a positive sign. Of course, people aren't always fully transparent, and there's no foolproof way to guard against that, but generally, when someone treats their ex with respect (taking into account of course the parameters of which it ended, as this might not always be warranted!) it speaks volumes about their emotional intelligence and integrity.

Shared values

While we explored shared values in the dating chapter as a foundation for forming connections (*see* p. 79), they're just as essential, if not more, when it comes to sustaining and nurturing those relationships over time.

Values shape what matters to us in day-to-day life and they affect how we act and behave. Psychological research shows that couples who share core values – especially values like honesty, empathy, mutual respect and caring for others (what some psychological studies call 'self-transcendence values') – tend to experience higher relationship satisfaction, fewer conflicts and greater emotional well-being.

So, if you're looking to lock someone in long term, you'll want to make sure at least a few of your fundamental values align.

If you're new to same-sex relationships then it's common to sometimes be blindsided with the idea that because you're both women, then you must think and feel roughly the same things, but unfortunately (sorry to burst the bubble), this isn't necessarily true.

We're all individuals with our own respective histories, experiences, hopes and fears and although you both might enjoy lighting a candle and watching Netflix together in the evening, you also need to figure out exactly *who* this person is underneath that.

If you can recognise similarities past the surface level between you (and more importantly enjoy and respect them) then this is a fantastic sign.

Being able to talk about mental health

The LGBTQ+ community is no stranger to mental health conditions. It's gotten to the point now that it's almost a rite of passage to have had at least a few first dates where you discuss what trauma you've experienced and what medication you're on to deal with it, before you're even on drink number two.

A lot of people in the queer community struggle with mental health complaints due to the nature of the coming out and acceptance process. Even if you haven't experienced many external hurdles from society, family or friends then you might have had internal battles that have weighed heavy along the way. Coming out (as we explored chapter 1) is a difficult process, with many ups and downs, and sometimes it takes a long time to process and accept things.

For young LGBTQ+ people in the USA (aged 13 to 24), '65% report having at least one diagnosed mental health condition', with anxiety, depression and ADHD among the most common. But it's not only a youth issue. Among LGBT adults aged 30 to 64, nearly 'half report symptoms of anxiety or depression, roughly 45% for anxiety and 40% for depression' – far above rates seen in non-LGBT peers.

So these conversations at the start of a relationship feel typical because, for many of us, our mental health is deeply intertwined with who we are, where we've come from and what we're carrying. It's highly likely that mental health complaints will show up in your relationship (either from yourself or others) so it's important to have open dialogue around them.

A great green flag is when someone is willing to share this information with you as your connection develops. It might be a really hard and painful thing to do, but in order to fully embrace and understand a person we need to know the full picture, so if someone is able to show you that vulnerability, then that deserves respect.

Equally, it's important to remember that vulnerability doesn't have to mean revealing everything all at once. Healthy relationships allow space for boundaries, and it's OK to take your time when opening up. You don't owe anyone your full story straight away: trust builds gradually and sharing parts of yourself should feel safe, not pressured. A good sign is when someone respects that process and allows you to share in your own time. Letting someone into your deeper layers is an intimate act, and doing so slowly, when it feels right, is not only valid, but also wise.

They have their own things going on

I simply cannot stress enough how much of a green flag it is if the other person you want to connect with has their own ambitions, goals and side quests that are *separate* to yours.

Often when we're new to dating women the idea of having both a partner *and* a best friend rolled into one can be a thrilling prospect but it can also mean that it's easier to lose sight of ourselves too.

It's tempting to treat your partner as you would a friend and invite them to every social gathering, include them in your hobbies and share your friendships, but remember, a healthy relationship is one where you can maintain your own identity as well as your shared identity as a couple. So if the person you're looking to deepen your connection with has their own interests and hobbies, and you do too, then it's a great basis for building not only a good relationship but a healthy, balanced schedule too.

I asked my community of queer women to weigh in on the green flags they look out for when dating women:

QUEER VOICES

'Warmth, humour, and emotional availability. Someone who communicates openly and makes you feel safe to be yourself.'

'Emotional maturity/intelligence, kindness, a passion for growth and understanding, respecting boundaries, a quick-witted sense of humour, thoughtfulness without being asked, effective communication, allows her inner child freedom to explore...'

'Is flexible and understanding when plans change.'

'Ability to communicate their feelings clearly, integrity, have attended/currently attending/open to attend therapy for personal growth and to challenge unconscious bias, and a shared sense of reality about the world.'

'If they have kids, a good relationship with their co-parent. Absolute nightmare if not.'

'Liking the same comedians is a big green flag. My partner and I have in-jokes from comedy, even if we never watched it together. We can both pretty much finish any sketch the other one starts!'

Good and consistent communication is the greenest flag

'Good and consistent communication is the greenest flag, and probably is the best way to determine if someone is emotionally available.'

'Look for someone who is aligned with your values. I'm very responsible so I started looking for someone who takes care of their space and their life.'

'Communication. Not being afraid to talk about hard stuff and work through differences. Being open-minded.'

'Someone who is kind – not just nice. Kind is a way of walking through the world. Someone who cares about what you have to say, how you feel, and is curious about you and how your mind works. Someone who notices the little things about you, even the things you don't even notice about yourself. Someone who wants to laugh with you and stick with you during the harder times.'

Attachment styles

Developed in early relationships but influenced over time by identity, environment and social messaging, our attachment style can strongly impact how we navigate our relationships, and especially ones that might be emotionally ambiguous or in the grey area.

For example, someone with an *anxious attachment style* (*see* p. 180) might become hyper-attuned to shifts in attention or affection, seeking clarity or reassurance the moment the connection feels uncertain. On the other hand, someone with an *avoidant attachment style* may withdraw or downplay their feelings, fearing the vulnerability of being seen or needing someone. When these dynamics play out between two people, especially in a space where the relationship hasn't been clearly defined, it can lead to confusion, miscommunication and emotional shutdowns that feel like rejection, even if they're not.

Research in attachment theory supports the idea that understanding our attachment patterns helps us build healthier, more secure connections. While most of this research hasn't focused specifically on queer women, recent studies have begun to explore how attachment intersects with queer identity, showing that marginalisation, minority stress and social stigma can further shape attachment patterns and emotional responses in intimate relationships.

So when something in the relationship feels 'off', it's not always about the other person: it may be about what both of you are carrying, consciously or not. Naming that can shift the dynamic, opening space for honesty, self-compassion and a more grounded understanding of what's really going on beneath the surface.

Attachment styles aren't fixed, and they're not personality traits: they're emotional responses, shaped by experience. With awareness, effort and the right support, they can shift and evolve.

Understanding your attachment style can offer powerful insight into how you connect with others. Because when you understand yourself, you relate with more clarity, and that's where real change begins.

If you're curious to dive deeper, a quick internet search will lead you to plenty of insightful articles and studies. To anyone looking to better understand themselves and their patterns, I'd recommend exploring this. In the meantime, here's a simple breakdown of different attachment styles to help you start exploring your own:

Secure attachment
(Rooted in consistent, nurturing caregiving)
People with a secure attachment style tend to feel comfortable with both emotional closeness and healthy independence. They're able to express their needs clearly, listen openly and trust in the stability of a connection without needing constant reassurance.

They usually grew up in environments where love was consistent, care was dependable and their emotions were met with acceptance rather than dismissal. As a result, they learned that relationships are a safe space, not something to fear or control.

In romantic dynamics, they're often emotionally available, supportive and comfortable with vulnerability. They can navigate tough conversations without shutting down or becoming defensive. They give love freely, and they receive it with ease, not because they've never experienced hardship or pain, but because they've learned how to regulate it without turning away.

Anxious (preoccupied) attachment

(Often shaped by inconsistent caregiving, sometimes present, sometimes not)

Those with an anxious attachment style often crave deep closeness but simultaneously fear being left behind. They tend to overanalyse situations, seek frequent reassurance and struggle with a sense of internal security in relationships.

This style typically develops in childhood when love and care were unpredictable: sometimes warm and available, sometimes cold or withdrawn. As a result, love became something to chase, rather than something they could trust would stay.

In queer dynamics, especially those in the grey area, this can look like constant overthinking, obsessing over what was said or unsaid, and clinging to any moment of intimacy as a sign of certainty. Anxiously attached people may blame themselves when things shift, thinking if they were 'better' or 'not as much', maybe the other person wouldn't pull away.

They don't lack emotional depth: in fact, they feel things deeply. But without tools to self-soothe, they can become overwhelmed by the fear of loss.

Avoidant (dismissive) attachment

(Usually develops from emotionally distant or rejecting caregivers)

Avoidantly attached people tend to value independence and self-sufficiency over emotional closeness. They often feel uncomfortable when others get 'too close' or when emotional expectations are placed on them, not because they don't care, but because vulnerability feels unfamiliar and unsafe.

This attachment style often forms in environments where emotional expression is discouraged or met with criticism. They may have learned early on that showing neediness led to rejection, so they adapted by not needing anyone at all, at least on the surface.

In queer connection, this can present as hot-and-cold behaviour, defensiveness or emotional unavailability. They may pull away when things start to deepen or seem to shut down in the face of intimacy.

Beneath the surface, many avoidant people long for connection, but the moment it becomes real, their internal alarm goes off, convinced that needing someone will only lead to disappointment.

Disorganised (fearful-avoidant) attachment
(Commonly linked to early trauma, loss or chaotic caregiving environments)

Disorganised attachment is often the most complex. It's a confusing blend of both anxious and avoidant tendencies, craving intimacy while simultaneously fearing it.

This style usually forms in childhoods where caregivers were sources of both comfort and fear, perhaps due to trauma, unpredictability or emotional volatility. These individuals never developed a consistent strategy for getting their emotional needs met, because the environment was too unstable to learn what was safe.

In relationships, especially queer ones where the stakes often feel higher, this can manifest as push-pull dynamics, reaching for closeness, then retreating just as quickly. These individuals may want connection deeply, but their nervous system is constantly on high alert, unsure whether love is safe or dangerous.

They often carry a deep fear of abandonment, but also a deep fear of being 'too much', 'too messy' or 'too broken'. As a result, they may sabotage intimacy, not because they don't care, but because the experience of closeness feels emotionally overwhelming and unpredictable.

Entering a long-term relationship with another woman

Getting past the early stages of dating and stepping into a longer-term relationship with another woman can be both beautiful and complex.

The spark is (hopefully) still there, and now you're on your way to building something deeper.

Your guards are down, you've likely seen each other in both good and messy moments, and the connection that once felt excitingly unknown now feels rooted and *real*.

But with that intimacy also comes vulnerability, and the possibility of warning signs becoming more apparent.

When someone really knows you – your habits, patterns, triggers and fears – it can feel exposing. And in queer female relationships, where emotional intensity often runs high, these deeper layers can stir things up in unexpected ways.

You might find yourselves navigating different attachment styles, unhealed parts of your past or internalised beliefs about what a relationship 'should' look like. You might also hit new levels of joy, closeness and comfort that surprise you, in the best possible way.

The journey can take many different turns.

So let's explore what tends to come up as a relationship deepens. From communication challenges and emotional triggers, to building healthier foundations and recognising patterns, what follows are some of the real-life dynamics that shape longer-term connection, and ideas for how to move through them.

Moving in together

One of the first steps you might take to deepen your connection with another woman is to merge your lives and potentially move in together, but it's important to remember that moving in isn't just a *practical* change; it's an *emotional* one too. So, if you're still in the early stages of dating, it's worth pausing to really reflect on what this step truly means, and whether you're genuinely ready for all that it brings.

Living with someone full time is very different from spending weekends together or going on the occasional trip. You're in each other's space constantly, and all the little quirks and habits (yes, even the annoying ones) come to the surface. Things like cleaning the toilet, sharing chores or picking up towels off the floor (yes women can do this too) can start to chip away at the 'hot and sexy' honeymoon energy. It doesn't disappear, but you may need to work more intentionally to keep it alive once you're sharing a home.

In one previous relationship, when we decided to move in together, the dynamic shifted quite dramatically in ways I hadn't anticipated. Our routines and expectations didn't align, tensions became more frequent, and aspects of day-to-day life together proved more challenging than I had imagined. It was an experience that showed me how much can change once you share a space. Sometimes you don't know these things before you take that step, but it reinforced the importance of understanding not only whether you work well together romantically, but practically too – and that those can be very different things.

That said, moving in together can also be deeply rewarding. It creates opportunities to grow as a couple, to communicate better, to build routines that suit you both, and to support one another in a more grounded, everyday way. Some people naturally thrive when they blend their lives; for others, it takes time, patience and a few 'domestic' conversations to find your flow.

It can all be a bit confusing. Without widespread examples or open conversations about what healthy queer relationships actually look like, it's easy to second-guess your feelings, to wonder if you're being too sensitive, too reactive or expecting too much.

It's also important to remember that even the healthiest couples go through rough patches. But challenges can offer opportunities for growth, deeper communication and stronger connection. And it takes time and self-awareness to understand the difference between a relationship that's evolving, and one that's undermining your well-being.

Warning signs to look out for

One of the most powerful lessons I've learned – from myself and others – is that your intuition matters, no matter who you're dating. If something doesn't feel right, it's worth listening to that inner voice. We're often quick to recognise when a job or friendship no longer serves us, but when it comes to romantic relationships, especially queer ones, where representation is still lacking, it can be harder to admit when things aren't working. Hope, love and denial can keep us stuck in spaces that don't nurture us.

That's why learning to spot warning signs and trust your feelings are such crucial steps. They're how you move towards the kind of connection that feels not only exciting, but safe, supportive and sustainable. So here are some of the more common warning signs and where things might get complicated, as well as some advice from me and the queer women in my community for how to recognise and potentially resolve them:

A breakdown in communication

Communication rarely breaks down all at once. It's not just one or two unresolved arguments: it's usually a gradual erosion that happens over time, often without either person fully realising it.

In many relationships, different communication styles are a key source of tension, especially when it comes to conflict. Maybe you express yourself directly and value getting everything out in the open, while your partner tends to shut down or withdraw when things get tense. One person might see directness as cold or harsh, while the other views avoidance as dismissive or emotionally distant.

Neither style is inherently wrong, they're just different.

But when those differences go unacknowledged or unaddressed, conversations can quickly become frustrating cycles of misunderstanding, where no one feels truly heard.

To prevent miscommunication from growing into resentment, it's important to recognise and respect your differences, while also finding common ground.

Building a communication style that works for both of you often involves compromise, patience and a shared willingness to better understand each other, not just in how you speak, but in how you listen.

Choosing to understand your partner is an active and ongoing decision that reflects growth and commitment in a healthy relationship. The willingness to learn about each other, whether it's about their feelings, needs or perspectives, is a powerful sign that the relationship is evolving and deepening, which in turn shows that both people are invested in nurturing the connection and growing together.

On the other hand, no matter how long you've been together, if you find yourself unable or unwilling to put in that effort, it can often signal that the connection is beginning to fade, or perhaps you're not in the right headspace to pursue the relationship at that particular moment.

Misaligned values and future goals

It's important to preface this by saying that you don't need to have *every single* value and future goal aligned with the other person (or people) that you are in a relationship with for it to be successful – but you do need to have *enough* in common that you can see eye to eye and carve out a future that feels authentic to you.

These values and future goals can also *change*. It would be naive to say that a relationship stays the same as time progresses. We all shift and change regularly as we learn more and experience more in life, but to maintain a healthy partnership with someone means growing *together* and working to complement each other as you evolve.

Unfortunately for a lot of people who enter into relationships, they fail to acknowledge this and assume that the other person will continue to stay the same, and that they in turn will too.

We're fed the narrative that the 'hard work' is finding and 'locking in' a person but really the hard work comes as time progresses, to ensure that you stay on the same page and continue to support each other's individual journeys as well as your shared one.

When your connection in a relationship deepens, so do the conversations.

What often begins with shared interests and surface-level aspirations can gradually shift to more complex discussions about values, long-term goals and what you want from life. Sometimes, over time, differences that seemed small at first can start to feel more pronounced.

Arguments or disagreements around values can emerge from the seemingly trivial, how to organise the home, what to buy at the grocery store, or from more significant topics, like children, finances or differing visions for the future.

Sometimes, the biggest misalignments aren't immediately obvious until months in, and they can leave one or both partners feeling uneasy, questioning whether the relationship is truly sustainable. Even when both people want to make things work, there can be moments when compromise simply isn't possible.

Deepening a relationship isn't just about closeness or shared excitement, it's about ongoing negotiation, honest reflection and recognising when your needs and boundaries might be diverging, even if it's hard to admit.

My biggest advice to anyone who is struggling with a misalignment of their values or goals in a relationship is to really take time to sit in your feelings and think about what you want. There are many tools on the internet (including a piece of work done by the VIA Institute where you can take a values survey to learn more about yourself), podcasts and books that will help you with this journey.

Another very simple activity could be to note down the qualities and values you admire and love about the people closest to you. It's very likely that what they already have is what *you* value too, as you've let them into your life.

When I look around, my closest platonic connections are hilariously funny, kind, honest, loyal and grounded. These (not surprisingly) are the traits I also exhibit, and in turn, look for, in a romantic connection.

It's also important to know that value misalignment doesn't always mean a relationship has to end. Sometimes growth can come from learning to understand and respect your differences, even if you don't fully share them. If you and your partner are both willing to communicate openly, compromise where it feels healthy, and stay curious about each other's perspectives, then that in itself is a sign of growth.

The key is noticing whether the relationship creates space for both people to evolve, individually and together, without one person constantly shrinking to accommodate the other. If that mutual space to grow exists, then misalignment might not be a roadblock, but rather an invitation to deepen your connection in new ways.

Failing to acknowledge mental health challenges

Struggling with mental health doesn't make someone a bad partner. The issue arises when those struggles aren't acknowledged or managed, and instead become a reason, or an excuse, to treat others poorly.

Everyone goes through difficult periods, and not every day will feel good. That's a normal part of being human. But when those tough periods start to feel unusually heavy or begin to impact how you care for yourself or your partner, it's worth checking in: are you both still showing up with each other's best interests in mind?

During mental health challenges, it's easy (and often unintentional) for someone to become inward-focused and less aware of how their behaviour might be affecting the dynamic. That doesn't automatically mean the relationship is broken or doomed but it might mean that, right now, it isn't functioning in a healthy or balanced way.

Open, honest communication is key, not just about what you're struggling with, but also about what you need. And while it's valid to want to support a partner through hard times, your own well-being matters just as much.

Seeking support for yourself – from friends, family or professionals – isn't selfish; it's necessary.

If the relationship starts to feel consistently one-sided, emotionally draining or manipulative, it may be time to reflect on whether it's still the right space for you. Compassion and care are vital, but they shouldn't come at the cost of your own mental health.

Shame and judgement

If, like me, you're someone who naturally leans into vulnerability – who opens up, shares honestly and connects deeply with others – you'll know it can be a beautiful strength.

For many of us, it's how relationships grow in meaningful and authentic ways. But as empowering as vulnerability can be, it can also come with risks, especially in environments where two people are joining together and mixing a range of their past, present and future anxieties, insecurities, and, often for the queer community, potentially traumatic experiences that can leave a lasting mark on how you care for yourself and others.

The wrong relationship can create dynamics that sometimes, we're simply not prepared for. There are many reasons why relationships can shift and change shape, but what can start off as a meaningful connection, full of mutual sharing, vulnerability and safety can sometimes descend into an environment that feels uncomfortable, critical and emotionally unpredictable. This shift can be rapid or quietly unfold over time and it can be an incredibly tough thing to navigate, especially if you're new to queer dating.

Experiencing emotions of shame, criticism and judgement isn't easy, but we must learn to recognise and unpack where these come from. Yes, it's important to recognise that our own behaviours are not always healthy, and that this might be contributing to the overall dynamic of a partnership, but we must also recognise that shame, guilt and anxiety can be placed *upon* us from others too – in the form of projection, envy or even insecurity, for example.

Shame, guilt and judgement are more than just uncomfortable feelings: they create a deeply embodied experience, that can feel like an attack on our character. Shame and guilt also live in the body. You might notice your chest tighten, your throat close up, your heart race or a sudden urge to shrink or disappear.

These aren't just passing emotions – they're physical responses to the fear of being seen as 'too much', 'not enough' or somehow unworthy.

When you've opened yourself up in a relationship, shared honestly and leaned into vulnerability, and that openness is met with discomfort, dismissal or used against you, it can leave lasting marks. What once felt like connection begins to feel like exposure. And over time, you may start to hide parts of yourself, pull back or build emotional distance as a form of self-protection.

This isn't just emotional self-preservation: it's a survival response. Psychological research shows that shame can lead to withdrawal, self-criticism, anxiety and even physical symptoms. It can make you question your worth and feel like a burden, even when the issue lies in the dynamic, not in you.

In healthy relationships, vulnerability is met with care. In the wrong ones, it can become a source of pain, not because you were wrong to be open, but because the space wasn't safe enough to hold it.

MY STORY

This is a headspace I know all too well, as in one of my previous relationships, I was made to feel deeply ashamed of who I was and like my presence was unwanted. It didn't always come through loud arguments or obvious fights; it often showed up in quiet criticisms, subtle digs, and a constant sense that I was always doing something wrong.

Over time, I began to question everything: my friendships, my work, my character, even whether the people in my life actually liked me or if I had imagined it all. I carried guilt simply for being myself.

It wasn't until after that particular relationship ended that I started opening up to friends, and only then did I begin to realise that what I had experienced had never been healthy.

Deep down, I knew I should have walked away sooner, but I was scared: scared of losing a relationship with someone I had come to depend on, scared of letting go of the life we had built together, and scared to trust my own intuition. Staying wasn't a simple choice, it was entangled with emotional attachment, hope for change, and the comfort of familiarity.

When judgement and shame are present, they can cloud your ability to make decisions and leave you dependent on situations or people that perhaps aren't healthy. I knew I had the capacity to leave, but I was paralysed by the fear that any choice I made would be wrong.

I never imagined I'd end up in a relationship like that. Even now, it feels surreal to say it aloud, because I hardly recognise the version of myself that stayed. But once I began to name the shame I'd carried, something shifted. The weight started to lift and I reclaimed the narrative on my own terms.

Over time I have found that the best way to combat and move through any cycles of vulnerability, shame, criticism and the complex emotions that can arise in relationships dynamics, is to educate myself.

Learning to recognise when relationships might enter this unhealthy zone is crucial to protecting your own well-being and mental health, and that is why I have provided examples of green flags and warning signs in this chapter, in the hope that these, too, will expand your toolbox and allow you to take a step back, assess and figure out the next steps that are right for you.

Final thoughts on warning signs

Warning signals go across genders. There is no difference between being on the receiving end of hurtful words and actions from a man than there is from a woman, and sometimes we overlook this.

Abuse doesn't have gender boundaries and as shocking as it can be to figure out, (especially if you're new to queer dating), women are also capable of hurting other women.

None of this is meant to discourage you from being in a relationship with a woman, but the more of us who become emotionally aware, the less likely we are to tolerate harmful behaviour if it arises from *any* gender.

It's also crucial to remember that sometimes not all the issues in a relationship stem from the other person: sometimes they may come from your own patterns as well.

That's why understanding yourself, knowing who you are and what you value is so important. It helps you recognise whether the words spoken carry any truth or if someone is gaslighting you – a huge warning sign, among many others, that might be signalling that your relationship is in trouble.

I asked queer women to provide input on what they believe are warning signs in a relationship: what they have experienced, look out for and try to avoid. These aren't to place shame or judgement on others but to illustrate what has caused real pain and hurt, and how you might be able to recognise some of these patterns in yourself or potential partners and make sure your relationship is grounded in emotional health and mutual respect. Here's what they had to say:

QUEER VOICES

'Inconsistency and lying are big warning signs for me!'

'If they kept me a secret, poor communication, lack of basic consideration of others or dismissing my feelings.'

'As with many things, it's based on experience. I had a girlfriend for a while who wanted me to buy her designer clothes, business-class flights, five-star hotels, etc. I kind of felt that she loved me for my money rather than for me.'

'If they are emotionally reactive, desire to control everything, treat others poorly, no growth mindset, actions that don't align with

words, poor communication, disregard the feelings of others or narcissistic traits!'

'Not understanding my commitment to my children or being jealous of that.'

'Someone who engages in a lot of projection and hasn't owned their own shit yet and isn't willing to be wrong or take accountability.'

'If they don't care about the world and humanity around them, that says a lot.'

'I really value taking time to heal from past relationships. Does she still live in her friend's guesthouse because she just got out of her last relationship? Run!'

Navigating outside pressure on your relationship

Like many LGBTQ+ women, I have been in relationships which faced external challenges that put strain on the relationship, particularly around familial acceptance.

Some of the comments made to me in previous relationships have felt far from appropriate, and whilst I always tried to understand where the discomfort was coming from, it was often difficult not to absorb the tension, and over time, those undercurrents added weight to the relationships I was part of.

If you find yourself in this situation then I'd just like to say that you are *really* not alone.

What's most important is staying united as a couple. At the end of the day, it's your relationship that counts, not outside opinions.

Here are some quick nuggets of advice on how to navigate that:

- Make sure you get on the same page about how you communicate with *each other* around family and how you plan to communicate as a couple *with* the family.
- Set boundaries and understand what will be tolerated and what won't.

- If your relationship isn't public then sit with yourself and ask yourself whether you're *really* happy being kept a secret (because as much as you hope that this will change, it might take a long time and even then there will likely still be hesitance and resistance to work through). Not every relationship needs to be accepted by the wider family, but if this is one of your values and non-negotiables, then it's important to understand and honour that, for your own happiness.
- If all of the above can't be done or causes misalignment and disagreements in your relationship then it might be time to consider whether this partnership is right for you.

And to show you're not alone in this, I also asked my community of queer women to add their advice around navigating tricky family dynamics:

QUEER VOICES

'My in-laws played a large part in the breakdown of my marriage. There was a significant lack of acceptance about their daughter being gay, and that I'd "taken her away". The best way I can see to navigate something like this is to have boundaries that protect both the relationship and your own identity.'

'It's important to listen to genuine concerns if done respectfully, but equally to stay strong and keep boundaries. Only you two know your relationship and what's best for you!'

Only you two know your relationship and what's best for you!

'I think weighing the benefits and consequences is important. My parents have been clear they are not supportive and I have accepted that I don't need to tell them, in order to live my lifestyle. I can find people who are accepting of my sexuality elsewhere. Trying to reveal it to everyone when it isn't to your benefit isn't a very good idea.'

'I once loved a woman who was not out to her parents. It was very destructive and erasing, but there were moments of humour. She

once told me her parents had enjoyed the film Brokeback Mountain. *I said I wasn't sure it was giving a particularly positive sense of how gay relationships generally turned out . . .'*

Questioning if the relationship is right for you

If you've ever felt a quiet sense of restlessness growing inside you, like something no longer fits, even if you can't quite name why, you're not alone.

Sometimes the earliest signs that a relationship isn't right don't arrive as loud warning signs, but as subtle shifts: a craving for space, a longing for independence or a sense that you're beginning to lose touch with yourself. These feelings can be confusing, especially if things look fine on the surface, but they're often the first internal signals that something is shifting.

For queer women, recognising these internal signals and the end of a relationship can feel especially difficult and emotionally layered. It's not always just about walking away from a romantic partner: it can mean losing your best friend, your closest emotional confidante, and in many cases, someone who's deeply woven into your wider social world.

Because many queer relationships are built within close-knit communities or friend groups, the emotional and social overlap can run deep, making the idea of leaving feel like pulling away from an entire part of your identity or chosen family. On top of that, societal narratives often frame queer love as rare, hard-won or something we should hold on to at all costs, so when things aren't working, there can be a quiet pressure to stick with it, even when it no longer feels right. That can lead to a lot of confusion, guilt and second-guessing.

You might not just be mourning the end of a relationship, but also the loss of a version of yourself that existed within it. All of this can make it incredibly hard to know when to stay and when to gently begin to let go.

It's natural to wonder how you'll stand on your own two feet again after leaning on someone for so long, whether they were your comfort, your home or simply the person you shared everyday moments with. But while connection matters, relationships also need intimacy (whether that's emotional, physical or both) to truly thrive. If that's missing, it might be a sign your deeper needs aren't being met.

Being single is often painted as a 'lonely' thing, but there's nothing lonelier than staying in a relationship that no longer feels right.

MY STORY

One summer, I found myself sitting cross-legged on a warm balcony in the middle of a thunderstorm (very dramatic, I know). I was on a shoot abroad and found myself having a rare moment of solitary reflection; a chance to truly sit in my thoughts away from the noise of the world around me.

I slipped on my headphones and scrolled through old playlists. My thumb hovered, then landed on an album I'd had on repeat a few summers earlier when I was single and dancing at a festival with friends.

As the music played, I felt something shift. It brought back a sense of freedom and familiarity, a reminder of who I was before life became heavier, and I realised just how far I'd allowed myself to drift.

It felt like stumbling upon a forgotten version of myself, and in that moment I saw the paradox clearly: how happy I had once felt, yet how bound and tethered I now was to the life I was living.

Sometimes it isn't just the fear of what life might look like without someone; it's the fear of failure, of what walking away might say about you, and what all the months, years, or even decades you invested were meant to amount to.

But the truth is, when you're in the wrong situation or relationship, you'll always feel a sense of disconnection. Sure, healthy relationships go through phases of uncertainty, but if you're living in a constant state of sadness, grief or longing for a different life, that's often your inner voice nudging you towards change.

That discomfort isn't weakness; it's your cue to be courageous and begin a new chapter.

I remember looking at the thunderstorm and the lightning that night and whispering under my breath, 'How is the world so completely *alive*, yet I feel so *dead*?'

I wasn't dead. I had so much life inside me, but I couldn't access it.

I had buried it beneath the weight of fear and silence, too afraid to be honest, too hesitant to be brave.

This is a moment many queer women know all too well – the uneasy space where your emotions no longer align with the relationship you're in, and deep down, you realise that something has to give.

This is just one example of how the moment of realisation can show up for you, but there are many others. To explore this further, I reached out to my community of queer women and asked them to share how they knew their relationship wasn't right, and when they recognised it was time to walk away:

QUEER VOICES

'When the relationship had run its course, it took a long time for my heart to catch up with what my head already knew. When I took my marriage vows (and even renewed them!) I meant every word. But if someone can't meet you where you are, projecting hope again and again only leaves you drained. So, I had to stop self-abandoning and choose myself.'

'When they ask you for something you know you can't give them. Like marriage or kids. These are fundamental needs that will not change – or usually don't. They are core incompatibilities and even though I loved them, they would probably be happier achieving what they want from life with someone else willing to be on that journey with them.'

'It was my ex-wife. We had been together around 12 years and married for two. We simply fell out of love and the intimacy was gone; it was just like being friends. It was mutual – we spoke and agreed we just didn't feel the same any more, and we should separate. It hit me months later though.'

Do not be afraid to make that change

'When I realised I was trying too hard to make it work, rather than letting things fall into place. It was sad, but clear.'

'Realising we had no way of effectively communicating without infuriating each other. Communication is so key and should be easy from the very beginning.'

'I wanted to break up with my ex for nearly a year but things kept getting in the way (family deaths, Christmas, birthday, etc.). Eventually I just ended it mid-argument. Which is probably a terrible time to do it, but it ripped the plaster off.'

'I realised I deeply loved my spouse, just as a best friend and safe space, and I wasn't in love with her. After past sexual trauma, I thought that best friendship and security was what love was, until I discovered I could have safety, friendship and desire for someone. It was painful and I will always feel guilt, but ending it was the right decision.'

'I knew it was time when it was too late. I was emotionally broken, numb and not myself. One day I just turned around and said, "I don't like the way you are treating me." After 16 years I had been slowly ground down. My advice is do not be afraid to make that change. Only good things can happen when you hit rock bottom!'

MY STORY

As the end of the relationship that started to unravel on the balcony became increasingly inevitable, I began to notice internal shifts in myself. I felt agitated in ways I couldn't always explain, craving time alone and willing my autonomy to return.

RELATIONSHIPS

What once felt like connection started to feel like constraint, and I felt like I was shrinking within a dynamic that no longer reflected who I was, or more importantly, who I was *becoming*.

But, like most things in my life, even a break-up wasn't straightforward without a little chaos. After a trip abroad, where I'd finally had the headspace to think clearly, I walked through the front door, dropped my bags, and prepared to deliver the news that I thought our relationship should end. Instead, however, I was greeted with something that I wasn't expecting – a large hamper – complete with a giant red bow and my name on top, sitting awkwardly on the countertop, waiting for me.

I stared at it for longer than felt normal for a basket of food. I wondered if I should eat some of it because I was jet-lagged and hungry or make a plan to donate it after I broke the news. I googled 'local food bank' but there didn't seem to be one nearby, so the hamper continued to sit there like a ridiculous showpiece, haunting me in the corner of my eye until intrigue gave way and I finally undid the ribbon.

I'm not sure exactly what I was expecting to find but what lay inside was the final validation for my decision to walk away. Wrapped up in a gigantic bow was a vast selection of all the foods I hated and couldn't, because of my bowel disease, consume. I picked up a jar of pasta sauce and laughed. How could someone I had been in a relationship with not know me *at all*?

The day after discovering the 'hamper of doom', we took a drive, in a last-ditch attempt to rekindle things. 'I think we should be honest with each other,' I said and the bomb was dropped. Making way for one of the most awkward break-ups I've ever experienced, which eventually involved pulling up in a car park, mutually agreeing that it would probably be best to go our own separate ways and then having to drive back for two (very long) hours in silence with one fantastic interlude at a motorway service station where we both went for a wee, before calling it quits.

How to navigate life after a break-up

Break-ups are never easy, but breaking up with another woman can bring its own unique kind of complexity. Whether the connection was long-term, intense, casual or complicated, the emotional terrain can feel especially layered. The intimacy, the shared vulnerability, the blurred lines between romance and friendship – it all adds to the weight of letting go.

In this section, we're going to explore what happens after the end. What it really feels like to move through heartbreak, grief and healing, and how, even in the middle of the mess, there's space for growth, clarity and rediscovery.

The time following a break-up can be incredibly challenging for a variety of reasons, from the raw pain of loss to the uncertainty of what comes next. It's a period filled with a whirlwind of emotions: sadness, confusion, relief and sometimes even guilt or doubt. Yet, despite all this difficulty, it also holds a unique and powerful opportunity for personal growth and deep self-reflection.

When a relationship ends, it forces you to pause and look inwards in ways you might never have before. It's a chance to do the inner work that you might not have realised you needed, to unpack your feelings, examine the patterns that played out, and gain a clearer understanding of what truly went wrong.

This process also allows you to realign with your core values, rediscover who you are outside of the relationship, and tune into your authentic self with more clarity and compassion. For many queer women, particularly if this is your first relationship with another woman, this period can feel even more intense and emotionally charged. But it's a time to honour your experience, learn from it and begin laying the foundation for healthier, more fulfilling relationships in the future.

> ### A note on the universe (because I'm a big believer)
>
> Sometimes relationships don't end because it was the wrong person, they end because the timing wasn't right. And if you're someone who believes in the bigger picture (as I do), it's comforting to trust that what's meant for you will always find its way back. If two people are truly aligned, life might pull them apart for a while, but that connection will endure. Time and distance won't weaken it: it will clarify it.
>
> The space between you will only affirm how much you miss and value one another.
>
> And if it turns out you weren't meant to be, that person won't resurface, or if they do, the healing you've done will be so complete, the moment won't carry the same weight it once did. It'll feel lighter and more neutral, like a chapter that closed for a reason.
>
> The universe works in strange but deliberate ways. And while we can't always control how things unfold, we can trust that the right people, at the right time, won't pass us by.

How to heal and grow

With time, I've come to realise that every break-up I've been through has actually been one of the best things to happen to me. Each one has pushed me to grow into the person I've always wanted to become, to understand my sexuality more deeply, and to meet people who have genuinely changed my life – people I'm certain I never would have crossed paths with if I'd stayed with those ex-partners. At the time though (even if you're happy to have ended the relationship) it can feel confusing and scary to start over. Having to rebuild your own identity outside of a partnership is terrifying, regardless of how you feel about the other person, so if this is you right now then I want to hold out a hand.

Emotions are f*cking tough. It takes bravery and courage to go through a break-up regardless of whether the decision was yours, the other person's or mutual.

While some of my previous relationships ended without leaving lasting scars, I've also experienced the sharp, raw pain of others, and I can fully empathise with how deeply break-ups can cut, especially in relationships between women. It's a kind of grief that's hard to explain, even harder to prepare for, and one that takes many forms depending on the relationship and its ending.

That's why, alongside sharing what I personally learned through the process, from a no-nonsense, practical place, I've also gathered insights and advice from others who've experienced break-ups with women in very different ways. Some were painful, some were mutual, some were even a little funny in hindsight, but each offers something valuable, and a reminder that every ending looks and feels different.

Here are my (and others') top tips on how to heal and grow following a break-up:

Fighting for someone to love you isn't right

Heartbreak for another woman can be challenging to understand, especially if you've shared such a close connection with someone that you considered not only to be a partner, but a best friend too. It can feel like losing your world and everything in it all in one fell swoop, and it can be incredibly jarring, emotionally draining and simply sad.

However, fighting for someone to love you, proving your worth or putting your own life on pause to see if they change their mind will only prolong the hurt.

When someone chooses to walk away from another person, it's an active *choice*.

When someone chooses not to make a decision, it's still a *decision*.

The best thing you can do in this period is let time give you the clarity you need to look at things in a *removed* rather than *reactive* light. Only then can you reflect on what truly happened, what went wrong and what you need to move forwards. This might be in the form of a conversation, an apology or a closure in another form.

Just remember, though, that you might not always get the closure or explanation you desire, so it's important to build the tools to cope if that's the case. Use this period to get clear on who you are and your values, wants and needs. It will help you to enter your next relationship (when you're ready) from a clearer headspace.

You can do this through self-reflective practices like journalling, listening to podcasts and watching social media content, or you could work with a therapist and coach who might help you to see things in a different light. Relationship counsellors are there for a reason, and you should never be ashamed to unpack your feelings as part of a healing journey. It's a healthy thing to do.

I also highly recommend laughter, time with friends and exercise. These might sound simple or even clichéd, but they are powerful tools for healing. Laughter reminds you that joy still exists, even in the midst of pain, and that you're still capable of feeling it. Spending time with friends brings comfort, perspective and a sense of belonging that can often feel lost after a break-up, especially if your ex was also your closest companion. And movement, in any form, helps shift stagnant energy and release the emotional weight we often carry in our bodies. You don't have to run a marathon or become a yoga expert – just giving yourself a chance to reconnect with your body can be grounding and empowering during a time that often feels anything but.

Remember, there *is* someone out there who will show up for you, care and respect you and you won't have to convince them to stay.

And who knows, if you're truly meant to be with the person you're currently separating from, time apart might only strengthen the bond between you, no matter how things eventually unfold.

Break-ups aren't linear

I'll never forget the first time I saw my mum after a particular break-up with an ex-partner. She held my shoulders with both hands, looked me in the eyes and said, 'It's good to have you back.'

Sometimes others can see the collapsing of something from afar, a long time before the realisation dawns on you.

My previous break-ups have gone in many different stages, including drinking a lot of wine and buying lingerie, to staying up all night in strangers' living rooms at parties where we watched the sun come up. One time a break-up included an interesting period where my favourite pastime was to vape in the bath while eating a packet of salami (which I personally still think is an *excellent* stress-reliever and way of processing heartbreak – although please don't vape, it's really not good for you).

The point is, it's OK to heal from a break-up in the way that feels right to *you* in the moment.

Some of us might prefer to be around friends and disassociate, some might take weeks to reflect on their own, and some people might buy a plane ticket the next morning and disappear like Julia Roberts for their own version of *Eat, Pray, Love*.

It's never *time* that helps us to heal but instead the shift of mourning what could've been to accepting what *is*.

A friend once said to me in passing, 'It's not about the *what-ifs*, it's about the *what-nows*' – which I will always love.

However you arrive at your point of peace is irrelevant, so long as you find your way there in the end.

Protect your peace

A lot of people ask me how long they should leave it before they talk to their ex again or enter a new relationship. There are no rules for this and only through learning to trust yourself and your intuition will you find the answer.

Some people like to block their exes on social media, avoid talking to mutual friends and pick up new hobbies to avoid crossing paths. All of this is totally wonderful stuff, but in the long run, if you really step back and look at it, it's not sustainable.

Blocking or muting someone on social media as a way to avoid them (as much as we want to deny it) is a sign that you still *care* (unless of course you have good grounds to!). Granted, it's a way to protect your peace, but at some point (especially if you're dating in closer-knit queer communities or friendship groups) you'll likely have to face the feelings of seeing or hearing about them again in some form.

Remember the opposite of love isn't hate: it's indifference.

You will know when you're ready to move on when you feel *indifference* towards a person. It's not about wishing them ill, or necessarily even wishing them well, but simply not thinking about them at all.

That's the place we should aim to reach when we look back on our previous relationships.

To recognise where things fell short, feel the hurt without being overwhelmed by it, and find a space for forgiveness, not because you owe it to anyone, but because you owe it to yourself to let go of the parts of your past that try to weigh you down.

This isn't about being the bigger person, it's about recognising what *you* need in order to move forwards.

To close on an empowering note, I reached out to my community of queer women, asking them to share their advice on navigating heartbreak, so together, we can find strength and hope moving forwards:

QUEER VOICES

'Time. It's the only true healer. And therapy. Lots of therapy.'

'I have had therapy for many years and this for me is what keeps me grounded. It does get easier. Fresh air, walking, gym, swimming – anything that gets your heart going in other ways.'

'Don't listen to depressing music, re-read the conversations/messages or stalk on social media!'

'Make a list of 50 things that you love about yourself and know that you can bring unapologetically to the table in your next relationship!'

'Get under another woman.'

'Stay busy! It feels like you're losing a friend as well as a lover. It's hard.'

Feel it full and don't rush past the pain.

'Feel it full and don't rush past the pain. Surround yourself with the people and passions that remind you who you are beyond the past relationship or love.'

'Surround yourself with other women. Gain advice and resonate with experience. Also, go do something that brings joy to your heart! Go to a festival, dance all night, go kayaking! Remember who you truly are.'

'Sit with the emotions for as long as it takes. Do the little things that give you comfort, get fresh air and try to eat healthily. But ultimately it's gonna take time, so give yourself permission to feel shit for a while.'

'Remind yourself that it is so fun to fall in love with a woman, and you have the opportunity to do that all over again.'

Final thoughts on relationships

Regardless of how the story ends, relationships are not just about finding someone to share your life with, they're also about growth.

Every relationship between two women is different. Some are intense and passionate; others are calm and steady. Some last a season; others unfold over a lifetime.

None of them follow a single formula, and no one version is more valid than another.

What makes these relationships so rich is also what can make them complex: their emotional depth, the intensity of connection and the ways in which we continue to show up, no matter how hard it can feel with vulnerability.

But remember this: at the end of the day, the most enduring and meaningful relationship you'll ever have is the one you build with yourself. So protect it. Prioritise it. Nurture it. And when the time comes to let someone in, choose the person who sees you clearly, who wants to grow alongside you, not as someone to shape or fix, but someone to stand beside, exactly as you are.

SEVEN

The grey area of love

What do you call that moment, when you're talking to someone, and all you can think about is kissing them? The way they hold themselves, the way their words land effortlessly, and the way you catch each other's gaze for just a second too long, like you both know what's coming next. A deliberate tension in the air, daring you to do something you shouldn't, so much so that it takes everything in you not to lean across the table, stop them mid-sentence, and whisper, 'God, just *shut up* and let me kiss you.'

[I took a sip of wine.]
'Are you going to kiss *me*?' my friend asked, trying not to laugh.
'You're an idiot,' I sighed. 'I love you, but not like *that*.'

What is the grey area?

If you'd asked me in my 20s to define the difference between love and friendship, I would've told you that it fits into two neat boxes: one for platonic, another for romantic. As if there were a clear hierarchy, like two tiers of an emotional subscription service.

As I've gotten older, though, I've realised relationships, especially between queer women, are rarely black and white. The lines blur, labels don't always fit and we often find ourselves in that hazy, undefined middle ground where friendship starts to feel like something more.

The grey area can show up in many different ways. Maybe one, or both of you is still exploring your identity. You might be single, or already committed to someone else. Perhaps you've talked about your feelings but can't quite name what they are. Or maybe you've been friends for so long that it's hard to tell whether these emotions are new, or whether they've simply been simmering quietly beneath the surface, only now becoming impossible to ignore.

For many women, this grey area is where attraction to another woman first becomes visible. A close friendship might deepen unexpectedly, and somewhere along the way, something shifts. Sometimes one woman is already grounded in her sexuality, while the other is still questioning, exploring, or beginning to recognise desires she hadn't allowed herself to fully feel. And in some cases, romantic feelings develop on both sides, yet the nature of the connection remains blurry, suspended somewhere between friendship and something more.

This ambiguous space can appear at any time, whether you're single or already in a relationship, often becoming the quiet turning point where you start to see each other, or yourself, differently.

In the grey area *hope* is everywhere – hope that the connection is mutual, that it might grow into something more, that your feelings are valid and shared. But *fear* lives there too – fear of misreading the signals, of damaging a meaningful friendship, of rejection, or of coming face-to-face with parts of yourself you aren't ready to confront.

When these feelings go unspoken and the relationship stays undefined, the grey area can become emotional limbo: disorienting, intense and sometimes painful.

And yet, it's often in that limbo where the deepest intimacy lives. That's why this chapter matters, because naming the in-between gives us a way to move through it with more clarity, honesty and care.

That said, I want to be clear: this section of the book isn't about defining what 'love' between two people means – not because it isn't worth exploring (there are plenty of brilliant books out there that do), but because the word itself is far too expansive, and means so many different things to different people.

What I really want to explore is the space where the connection between two women grows complicated and doesn't quite fit into a neat category. What it looks like, how it feels, why you might find yourself there and, most importantly, how to start making sense of it all.

For the sake of this chapter, I'm calling this space the *grey area*. (Side note: there is a book called *The Grey Zone* about the space between life and death, so just to clarify, this isn't *that!*)

It's a space we don't talk about nearly enough, and I think it's time we did. So, take a deep breath – we're about to go somewhere real:

- Why the grey area is so common
- Why and how women bond the way we do
- Why it can be hard to define a connection
- How to start making sense of whether what you're feeling is platonic, romantic or somewhere in between
- What can happen when things are left undefined
- How to find clarity, whether that means moving forwards with someone, stepping away or simply understanding yourself a little better

And before we begin I think it's important to note that finding yourself in the undefined grey area with another woman can happen at *any* stage, before you come out, during your journey, or even long after. Sometimes you're the one in the grey area, sometimes she is, and sometimes it's both of you. Being in this space is rarely linear, often hard to navigate, and, like many relationships in the sapphic world, doesn't follow a clear script. And that's exactly why I've chosen to write about it.

Yes, it's a lot to unpack, but unpack it we shall, because, dear lord, it's needed.

Why is the grey area so common for queer women?

Before we dive in, let's get one thing straight: most of us aren't.

Sexual fluidity in women, especially as we get older, is far more common than people realise, and *definitely* more than we talk about.

We often laugh about 'late bloomers' or 'switching sides', but beneath the humour is something real. Women's sexuality is fluid: it shifts and evolves, shaped by biology, psychology and cultural conditioning. Finding this out can be freeing, but it can also be unsettling. It might upend long-held beliefs about who you are or complicate a friendship you deeply value.

Research shows that a significant number of women experience same-sex attraction without adopting labels like bisexual or lesbian. For example, the National Survey of Sexual Attitudes and Lifestyles found that of the 11.5% of women who reported same-sex attraction, only 2.4% of women in that survey self-identified as lesbian, gay or bisexual.

Similarly, *The Irish Times* Sex Survey revealed that '45% of younger women aged 17–34 reported being attracted to another woman', despite still identifying as heterosexual.

In other words, many women acknowledge their feelings but don't see them as central to their sexual orientation, creating a growing grey area between attraction, identity and action.

And this grey area doesn't just exist in theory: it's something I see reflected constantly in real life. I hear from women all the time, through my social media platforms and private messages, who are grappling with feelings they never expected to have.

Many are in long-term relationships or marriages with men yet find themselves navigating unexpected feelings for another woman. And this isn't a new phenomenon. In fact, a 1985 study revealed that 47% of married bisexual women were 'somewhat aware' of same-sex attraction before their heterosexual marriage, but were much less likely to have thought of or identified themselves as queer, even though their feelings for women often grew stronger during or after the marriage.

The words vary, but the themes are always the same:

'I know I shouldn't be saying this because I love him – but I also love *her*.'

Their messages are filled with panic, guilt, longing and confusion, and nearly all of them end with a version of the same sentence:

'I don't know what to do. I feel like I'm on my own with this.'

But the reality is that so many women have been there. You might be one of them or you might find yourself in a grey area with someone who is struggling – either way, you're *definitely* not alone.

To shed more light on this complex experience, I asked queer women to share what it feels like to realise you're attracted to another woman, especially if you're already in a relationship and fighting complicated feelings or have recently begun exploring your sexuality. Their stories reveal a mix of emotions that many women go through but rarely talk about openly:

QUEER VOICES

'I genuinely didn't realise I was queer until I was in my mid-20s – by which time I had been married to a man for five years. I grew up in conservative evangelical Christianity during purity culture, which meant my sexuality was incredibly repressed.'

'I think a part of me always knew I liked women but didn't understand that I was feeling attraction towards them because that's not how I was taught attraction was meant to feel. It wasn't until my mid-20s that I realised my curiosity about women was something more. It wasn't so much an immediate revelation but this slow burn of connecting the dots that helped me see just how queer I really am.'

'I once told a friend, "If I were into girls, I'd totally date her." It was a joke. But looking back, I really wanted to!'

'Honestly I thought we were just really good friends. We were always texting and talking (clue should have been the goodnight texts!) and I just remember thinking, "I wish my partner understood me like she does." I didn't even realise I was in love with her until she mentioned she was going on a date with someone and it made my stomach flip.'

'I met this woman on a night out with friends. I knew she was gay, and I'd always been curious about being with another woman. I had a boyfriend then, so I thought chatting to her was completely safe. But after a few drinks we ended up back at her place making out. I just remember how soft her lips were! My boyfriend and I stayed together for another six months after that (I think he found the whole thing a turn-on) but he's the last guy I ever dated, put it that way!'

'We were messaging constantly. I'd delete our conversations before my partner got home. Nothing happened, but I knew I was emotionally somewhere else, and at the time that really scared me.'

'For me it started with shared playlists and long voice notes that felt more intimate than texts to my boyfriend. I remember lying in bed listening to her laugh on loop and thinking, God, I'm in trouble. But it didn't feel wrong – it just felt confusing.'

'I was in my friend's hot tub when she unexpectedly straddled my lap, wrapped her arms around my neck and locked eyes with me. Decades of buried feelings that I might be gay came rushing to the surface.'

'I'm bi but have been married to a man for around 10 years. I met this woman through my friend's book club; we bonded over what we were reading and something about the way she looked at me just landed. We were friends for a while until I eventually told my husband about her and that I was developing feelings. I wasn't sure what it meant for us but I didn't want to lie. To his credit, he didn't freak out, he just said, "We'll figure it out together." That conversation was the start of us opening things up and communicating in a way we actually never communicated in before. We're both a lot happier now. It's been a bit wild, but so worth it!'

So, why is it that women's sexuality is generally more fluid than men's? Why does it often become even more fluid as we get older? And how can all of this lead to finding yourself either in the grey area yourself or interested in someone who (albeit perhaps unintentionally) places you there?

Psychologist Lisa M. Diamond's groundbreaking longitudinal study found that 'roughly 30% of women reported shifts in their sexual identity over time', highlighting just how fluid female sexuality truly is.

Experts like Diamond have argued that female sexuality is inherently more flexible, influenced by both biology and culture.

Biologically, women's sexual responses tend to be less fixed than men's. Instead of being driven purely by physical attraction, women's desires are often closely linked to emotional connection and the context they're in. This means feelings of attraction can be more fluid and influenced by *who* we're with and *how* we emotionally relate.

As explored in previous chapters, society plays a big role in shaping how women experience their sexuality. From a young age, girls and women often face pressures and expectations that discourage them from openly exploring, or even acknowledging, same-sex feelings. These pressures can come in many forms: the assumption that heterosexuality is the 'default' or only acceptable orientation, the fear of social rejection or judgement, cultural or religious teachings that label same-sex desire as wrong or sinful, and the lack of visible role models who openly embrace fluid or non-heteronormative identities.

Because of this, many women push those attractions aside or don't fully recognise them until later in life, when they feel safer or freer to explore what they're really feeling.

And on the topic of time: life changes. Shifting priorities, growing self-awareness and evolving social circles open the door to new experiences and a deeper reflection on who you are and what you truly want. More and more women are waking up to their own happiness, realising they don't have to live by others' expectations and as we get older, those external pressures tend to carry less weight. There's more room for self-acceptance, more time for reflection and less hesitation about putting your needs first and because of this, previously hidden or unacknowledged attractions can start to surface.

Why women bond deeply (and why it feels so real)

Connection between two women goes deep for many reasons: we're talking bonding hormones like oxytocin, social brain wiring that favours emotional closeness, evolved survival strategies and centuries of women turning to one another for comfort, resilience and strength.

But for queer women, this platonic connection can often have a subtle and silent romantic overlap...

We all know the energy: the way a friendship starts out feeling like a safe place, where you're unfiltered, share private jokes and late-night talks go on and on, and the world narrows down to just the two of you. It's safe and comforting, but there's always an undercurrent, something hot and a bit charged that makes you wonder if it *might* mean more.

It's what I like to call the dangerous sum of safety + excitement and it equals the kind of connection that doesn't come around often but when it does, it's impossible to ignore.

For many queer women, no matter what stage of the identity journey you're on, this kind of deep, emotional and often physical attraction can be one of the first real experiences of true *vulnerability*. Of fully being seen and known. It can feel like someone finally holding a mirror up to the parts of you you've buried, dimmed or hidden, whether out of fear, shame or simply not knowing they were there to begin with.

That's why understanding how and why women bond so deeply is important. If we can recognise the *foundation* of that connection, we might also be better equipped to understand when it crosses into something more.

So let's unpack it.

1. Patriarchy basically forced us to rely on each other

For centuries, patriarchal systems have done their best to isolate women, through marriage customs, inheritance laws and the good ol' 'your place is in the home' ideology. Women were pushed into domestic spheres, stripped of power and cut off from public life. But instead of crumbling, women built their own underground economies of care, emotional support, child-rearing and community organising.

Think of it as survival through solidarity.

So, when your connection with another woman feels *necessary*, not just *nice*, you're not imagining it. It *was* essential. And in many ways, it still is.

2. We're literally wired to 'tend and befriend'

While men are more likely to go into fight-or-flight mode under stress, research shows that women are biologically inclined to respond by nurturing and connecting. It's called the 'tend-and-befriend' response, and it's thought to have evolved as a way to protect offspring and build alliances.

So when you're mid-crisis, hiding under a duvet and instinctively texting your bestie (or perhaps someone you wish was in bed with you) you're tapping into an ancient, evolution-approved coping strategy.

3. Oxytocin crashes the party

You know that warm, fuzzy, slightly floaty feeling you get after a good hug or a vulnerable conversation with a female friend? That's oxytocin, the 'bonding hormone', doing her thing. Oxytocin gets released during emotional intimacy, cuddles and yes, even during shared crying sessions. Oestrogen boosts oxytocin's effects, which means women are especially susceptible to forming deep emotional ties after intimate moments.

So if you're wondering why one vulnerable chat made you feel wildly connected to someone ... this is why.

(Oxytocin is also released in abundance during sex, just FYI, so you can only imagine the chemistry floating around between two women after that.)

4. We've got emotional radar, and we're using it

Women are generally more emotionally expressive and more likely to engage in mutual self-disclosure (aka deep chats, vulnerability, emotional unpacking) than men. Whether it's due to socialisation, biology or both, we're often more attuned to the emotional cues and signals of those around us. This makes our connections layered, nuanced and, at times, borderline telepathic. And when two emotionally fluent people lock in like that? Sparks can fly, even if you're not calling them that yet.

5. Because 'friends first' is actually the default

Did your feelings start off as 'just friends' and then kind of ... spiral? You're not alone. Research shows that 68 per cent of romantic relationships begin as friendships, and if you identify as LGBTQ+, that number jumps to a whopping 85 per cent.

Even more interesting? Those friendships tend to simmer for almost two years before turning romantic. So if you're in that 'Are we just really close?' phase, you're not in limbo – you're often exactly where a lot of sapphic love stories begin.

So when you line up the biology, the emotional fluency and the centuries of women relying on one another for connection and survival, it starts to make sense. Female friendship isn't just 'girlhood': it's powerful, intimate and often layered in ways that until we analyse it, we don't fully recognise.

And even when we *do* understand why the connection feels so strong, that doesn't mean we suddenly have the language to name it. Sometimes it's not a question of simply 'Do I fancy her?' but more about what being around her *does* to you, and all of this is a space that queer women know well.

I asked my community of women to share their own stories: what it felt like to find themselves in that grey area with another woman, where the lines weren't clear, but the feelings were very real:

QUEER VOICES

'I had a situation with a girl who was married but was very flirty towards me, which I found confusing. I think on her part there was a bit of emotional cheating even though nothing physical happened between us. It was a very intense six months of messaging daily and going to the gym together and then she moved to a different part of town and I basically got ghosted.'

'She was my friend from work. We kissed after a Christmas party but she wasn't out and didn't think it meant anything. We had a back-and-forth emotional relationship for months until I decided I couldn't do it any more. I really liked her, but it wasn't going anywhere and it was driving me insane. It was really sad because I saw her every day at the office, but I had to cut contact or else I would have never moved on!'

'I was in the grey area with a married woman who was also my boss's boss's boss. It began as HR support during my ill health, then blurred into mentorship, friendship and a complicated affair that swung between love declarations and "just friends". It was intense, messy and a painful example of how queer friendship and romance can blur.'

'She was my co-worker and super confident. I thought I was just really inspired by her. I'd go home and tell my husband how clever she was! We had an emotional back-and-forth for months; I knew she liked me. One night after work she said, "Can I kiss you, or are you going to pretend this isn't happening?" I didn't pretend. I didn't end my marriage because of it, but it was the catalyst for me realising I *actually had feelings for women and needed to have a conversation both with myself and my partner!'*

'I was in the grey area with a woman who had a girlfriend. I always knew she wasn't happy. She'd reach out to me a lot. At first I thought it was hot, like this secret little thing we had, but the more that it went on, I realised I was being used as her emotional outlet. It was confusing because I liked her, but she wasn't being fair or honest to herself or me!'

The testimonials reveal how complex and layered these connections between women can be: full of attraction, confusion, hope and hesitation.

For many, it's not a straightforward story of friendship turning into love or something clearly defined: it's a back-and-forth, a space where feelings flicker between deep friendship and something more, often leaving us unsure of what to call it or how to move forwards.

For many queer women, the most real and intense connections often happen outside of scripts and expectations. That doesn't make them any less important: it just means they are yours to define.

Not every connection has a tidy label or a clear path, and that's OK. But I'm going to try to put words to it, to explore what that feeling of being in the grey area really is, what it means and why it feels so important.

Because, unsurprisingly, I've been there too.

MY STORY

When I first met Kate* I knew I wanted to be her friend. She was smart, funny and effortlessly pretty, with an energy that felt strangely familiar – like we were already halfway through a conversation that hadn't yet begun.

It wasn't just her laugh, her kindness or the way she treated every random thought I blurted out, as if it actually mattered, but the sum of it all – the way she made everything feel lighter, brighter and more alive, simply by being in the room.

Our friendship started the way most friendships do. We swapped films and TV shows, made up stupid inside jokes and complained about people we didn't like. But underneath, as time went on, I had a growing sense that it was beginning to matter more to me than it probably should.

I couldn't explain it then and, I still struggle to explain it now. I just wanted her time, her stories, her closeness, the part of her that had slipped so easily into my life, yet was already shared with someone else: her partner.

(Not exactly ideal when you're developing feelings for someone.)

Still, it didn't take long to notice that maybe I wasn't the only one quietly aware of what was happening. One night, we exchanged a look that friends rarely do and the unspoken question of *Are you thinking what I'm thinking?* suddenly felt too ridiculous to ignore, because, well, we absolutely *were*.

After that, I had no idea what to do with myself. Should I bow out gracefully? Lean in and risk total chaos? Or just have a quiet emotional breakdown? None of those sounded particularly appealing, so instead I did what I knew best: downed more Chardonnay, ignored the dynamic unfolding in real time and tried desperately to think about something deeply unsexy, like buying bin bags or filing my tax return. Anything to distract myself from how wildly inappropriate it felt to want someone who wasn't mine, yet who also seemed to want me too.

But you can only avoid something real for so long, and before I realised it, we were becoming part of each other's days in ways that wouldn't have made sense to anyone else.

She'd tell me off for stealing food, then nudge the plate towards me, so I could carry on. We never ran out of things to say, and the way she'd sometimes glance across at me and smile, thinking I wasn't watching, always made me smile too. That kind of intimacy is rare, and I knew it even then.

Looking back I don't think anyone 'fell', we just met somewhere in the middle. She found little ways to reach out, asking my opinion on the smallest things, and I'd text back just to see how her day had been. It felt effortless, the way we wanted to know each other.

We tried to pretend nothing had changed, after a moment that shifted things between us, but it had. Everything that followed carried the same unspoken question: *What do we do with this now?* There was no tidy answer, so the uncertainty became part of it – a sort of shared understanding that whatever it was, it mattered. And so we carried on, in the grey area between friendship and something more, because letting it go didn't feel right.

Often, we don't have a playbook for what to do when a connection like this hits us out of nowhere. I wasn't looking for it, but there it was: confusing, conflicting, and annoyingly hot.

And that alone was enough to shake everything up.

Maybe this story resonates with you, or maybe your experience looks completely different. There are countless reasons you might find yourself in the grey area; some will feel familiar, others entirely new. But the real question isn't how you got here, it's what you do now that you've arrived…

How to define whether you're in the grey area with another woman

So what do you do when you find yourself in that space with someone, where it's clearly more than friendship, but not quite something you can name? We've been taught how to be emotionally close with other women – how to care deeply, how to share affection without it needing to be romantic – but many of us were never taught how to recognise when those same feelings start to shift.

Defining what *kind* of connection you're feeling can be hard (sometimes even after having a conversation around it), but if you dig deeper you'll eventually find the subtle signs and moments that will give you the answer that you've been looking for.

To explore this more deeply, I've collected stories and advice from my community of queer women, alongside my own take on signs, moments and experiences, to help you start actually figuring out where your connection might sit. This isn't an exhaustive or definitive exploration – it's more like a guide to spark your own reflection about what different types of connection can look like.

Is it connection or intimacy?

Women are naturally curious about each other's lives; we go deep. We want to know who our friends are dating, what TV shows they're obsessed with and exactly what they added to that pasta dish to make it taste so good. We ask because we *care*.

But when it's just friendship, that care tends to have a ceiling, an emotional limit that romantic connection often surpasses.

When we look at the early stages of a relationship between two women who are attracted to each other, on a surface level, the conversations and topics appear to be quite similar to any close friendship, but if you look a little closer, you'll start to notice signs of something deeper – a unique emotional bond known as *intimacy*.

The *Oxford English Dictionary* defines intimacy as: 'closeness; familiarity or friendship; a detailed knowledge of a person; private and personal.' But intimacy goes beyond simple closeness. It's born from meaningful interactions, the frequency with which you share those moments and the effort both people put into being emotionally available to give and receive care. The Interpersonal Process Model of Intimacy expands on this, defining intimacy as 'A process in which one person expresses personal, self-relevant information (thoughts, feelings) to another, and the other responds in a way that makes the speaker feel understood, validated, and cared for.'

While *connection* is about discovering someone's interests and creating shared experiences, *intimacy* is about depth, vulnerability, trust and a willingness to be truly seen.

When I think of intimacy between any two people (regardless of gender or sexuality) I think of sex, or at least I did – until I learned that there's a hell of a lot more to becoming intertwined with someone than making out in your underwear to a Spotify playlist.

Intimacy shows up in *all* areas of our lives. It can be emotional through vulnerability, flirting and laughter or it can be physical through kissing, holding hands or, as just mentioned, playlist sex. It could be intellectual through thoughtful conversations, being creative and curious together or it could be experiential through navigating challenges or shared moments that push each of you out of your comfort zones.

All relationships carry some level of intimacy. But when you truly let someone in, you create a bond that transgresses friendship, a connection that reveals a deeper part of yourself – one you trust each other to see and hold with care.

For queer women, where emotional closeness is already deep and nuanced, reaching this kind of profound intimacy usually means something more than friendship. It's often not an accidental kind of closeness – it's intentional and purposeful.

I asked queer women what intimacy with another woman means to them:

QUEER VOICES

'For me, intimacy is about being fully seen and feeling safe enough in that connection to lay myself bare. Friendship offers steadiness, but with love there's an undercurrent of longing – when her presence stirs something in me that shifts the connection into desire.'

'Intimacy is vulnerability and letting someone see you fully. I usually know it's more than friendship for me quite quickly. I.e. Am I thinking about them constantly and do I want to take their clothes off? I've not been a regular "friends to lovers" experiencer.'

Intimacy is vulnerability and letting someone see you fully.

'I think if you have to question yourself about whether a connection with someone is friendship or love, then you may be leaning closer to the second one than you think.'

'If you're getting each other off, or trying to get to that level, that's intimacy. It's more than a friendship and you need to vocalise that!'

'I adore intimacy in every relationship because I love when vulnerability and safety coexist. What differentiates friendship from becoming something more to me is reciprocal longing to explore everything about the other person.'

'Sex! I personally can't have sex casually so if I slept with my friend, there would be serious conversations about what we both want.'

Mirroring

Mirroring shows up in all types of relationships, no matter your sexuality, but it tends to be especially strong in emotionally intense connections – something often seen between two women who share a romantic or more-than-platonic bond.

At its core, mirroring is when we subconsciously imitate another person's behaviours, speech patterns or preferences. It's something humans naturally do to build trust and closeness. It's the perfect illustration of what it means to become so emotionally entwined with someone that *part of them becomes part of you*.

In friendships between women, mirroring might look like sharing mannerisms, inside jokes, body language or gestures. But in deeper, emotionally charged connections, it often goes even further: aligning personal style, music tastes, matching food habits or even syncing menstrual cycles (although many studies have challenged the validity of this phenomenon).

While platonic relationships absolutely involve mirroring, the depth and frequency with which it happens between women navigating something more than friendship is often strikingly more pronounced.

But it's less about *how* you mirror each other, and more about what it reveals: a sense of unity, shared experience and emotional intimacy that's hard to fake. And really what's more beautiful than two people who can't get enough of each other, slowly integrating pieces of one another into their daily lives?

It's a bit like penguin pebbling – the ritual of offering smooth stones to one another as a sign of affection and nest-building. In the same way, humans exchange ideas, gestures, jumpers and playlists. The active choice to bridge the gap between where one person ends and the other begins is often a quiet sign that we want to be closer.

We *match* with our friends.

We *merge* with the people we love.

Why flirting is hard to resist (especially when you're into her)

Flirting isn't just playful, it's hardwired into us. Studies on nonverbal communication show that we send tiny signals called 'contact-readiness cues' like prolonged gazes, lean-ins or subtle smiles to signal openness to deeper connection. These actions are so universal they show up across cultures, genders and sexualities as primal ways to indicate romantic interest.

So what changes when the flirting is *not just friendly*?

I'm a cheeky person. I often throw down lines for my friends. It's playful, everyone feels good and we laugh about it. It is in its very essence *innocent* because I have no desire to act upon my flirting. I don't fancy my friends; my intention is platonic.

When two women like each other though, we break the rules of 'friendly flirting'. Time ceases to exist, eye contact lasts longer and lines hit heavier. Hearts race, boundaries are crossed and we let them – because this is no longer just friendship.

Any self-aware person knows what they're doing when they flirt. We don't willingly place ourselves in these types of situations unless we're not a little bit curious about the outcome.

Context and intention make all the difference. With friends, flirting feels light and safe. But when attraction is real, flirting shifts. It becomes more about curiosity and possible reciprocation; it's a subtle test of, 'Are you feeling this too?'

What happens when two women intentionally flirt?

When two women flirt with each other, the interaction often unfolds through subtle, indirect and predominantly nonverbal cues rather than the kind of overt verbal or physical advances we might see in typical heterosexual flirting.

This style of communication includes behaviours such as sustained eye contact, mirroring each other's body language, and sometimes, consensual touch.

In same-sex interactions, women often engage in shared laughter, playful teasing and synchronising gestures to build emotional intimacy and connection. Research on body language and behaviour shows that 'sincere flirting' for females involves laughing and smiling more frequently, reflecting an emphasis on warmth and emotional connection.

These behaviours exemplify what researchers call 'affiliative flirting' – a form of flirting characterised by friendliness and emotional rapport rather than explicit or goal-oriented signals. Affiliative flirting serves as a way for women to gauge interest and create a comfortable social environment.

Flirting can blur the lines between friendship and romantic interest, especially with another woman. It becomes more than friendship when there's emotional intensity, physical attraction, frequent one-on-one communication or if you think about her often and prioritise her emotionally.

So reflect on the following:

- **Check your feelings** – Do you get butterflies or feel jealous when she's with someone else, especially if she's flirting with them?
- **Notice your behaviour** – Are you going out of your way to impress her or spend time with her?
- **Imagine telling someone else about your bond** – Would it feel like a crush?

If the answer to several of these is yes, then your flirting likely has deeper emotional or romantic roots.

Communication

The frequency of communication between two women who like each other is almost *ridiculous*. Not in a judgemental way, more in a comical way: how completely blind we can be to someone's interest levels and effort when we're caught up in the thrill of talking to someone we're attracted to.

I've had friends experience constant communication, their phones blowing up from first thing in the morning until they hit the pillow at night, sometimes for weeks or even months – yet they still ask me the same question:

'Do you think she likes me, Rosie? Or do you think we're just *friends*?'

This constant communication makes a lot of sense when you consider the science behind it. When we fancy someone, our brains release dopamine and oxytocin, chemicals tied to pleasure and bonding, pushing us to seek connection and reassurance through ongoing contact.

For queer women, this is often intensified by the social complexities and invisibility we experience in heteronormative spaces. Without clear cultural scripts for flirting or dating, we rely heavily on the subtleties – texts, calls, shared laughter or memes – as a way to interpret interest, build trust and foster emotional closeness.

So those endless messages aren't just noise – they're the brain's way of trying to define and solidify a connection using words and subtle cues.

Women attracted to each other are also on a fact-finding mission! The communication can be frequent, detailed and borderline journalistic.

On the surface, conversations between two friends and two romantically interested women might seem similar, but it's the *why* that sets them apart.

'*Why* did you break up with your ex?'

'*Why* is sunset your favourite time of day?'

'*Why* are you feeling down?'

That 'why' is an invitation to a deeper understanding.

It doesn't matter what the questions are about: what matters is that this person is trying to soak up every part of you. Your 360. Your life story, hopes, fears, desires and flaws – your *everything*.

I'd never really had to dig into my dating history or question why I'm drawn to certain people, or what I actually want from a relationship, until women began showing interest in me that went beyond friendship. Suddenly they became like columnists on a mission to expose what turns me off, and more importantly, what turns me on.

The reason behind their questioning was simple: to learn how to show up as someone who does less of what gives me the ick and more of what gets me into bed. (Spoiler: it usually involves red wine and someone who knows how to put me in my place. Bonus points if you remember the sound of dial-up internet.)

They wanted to understand me more deeply than most, to get inside my inner circle and my inner world. That desire makes all the difference.

Sure, rolling conversations peppered with images, videos, voice notes and goodnight texts can happen between friends, but context matters. Continual communication is a form of effort that takes things a step further.

If I'm texting you day and night, I can assure you: I don't want to be your friend. I want to be under you (or on top; your choice.)

What happens when you feel stuck in the grey area?

For many queer women, the emotional grey area between friendship and romance can feel both comforting and deeply destabilising, and more often than not we reach a point where we feel stuck, static and unsure of how to move forwards.

Staying in the grey area offers closeness without pressure, and intimacy without the risk of rejection. But over time, that lack of clarity can become emotionally exhausting. Our brains are wired to seek definition and closure, and when that doesn't come, we can find ourselves spiralling into cycles of hope, doubt and sometimes even quiet heartbreak.

This ambiguity is often amplified for queer women, who grow up without clear cultural scripts for same-sex connection, and with the internalised belief that love, for us, is rare. When society has conditioned you to believe that you might never find the kind of love you're looking for, letting go of something that feels like it becomes even harder.

It's not just the person we fear losing: it's the possibility they represented.

For those who *can* muster up the words, we can try to address the feelings head-on, seeking clarity or defining the relationship. But queer women often face unique challenges here: societal invisibility, internalised doubt and a lack of how to phrase how we feel about navigating desire outside of heteronormative frameworks. Even naming the connection can feel risky or uncertain. And sometimes, even when the truth is spoken aloud, it doesn't lead to resolution – it simply confirms that the feelings are real.

Other times, the connection fractures. The grey area collapses, and neither friendship nor romance can be sustained. For queer women, who often have smaller, more intimate networks, this kind of loss can feel seismic.

These bonds may represent more than just romantic potential: they can be trusted spaces, places of happiness, and reflections of how we want to be seen and understood and the grief that follows is often ambiguous, unresolved and profound.

Psychologically, this limbo can keep our attachment systems activated long after the last message is sent or conversation closed, and even though walking away can become an act of self-preservation – a way to honour our own emotional boundaries when clarity, care or reciprocity is no longer on offer – these are not casual losses. They cut deep, precisely because they held so much meaning in the first place.

MY STORY

It was late May when I found myself sharing dinner with a new friend at a neighbourhood restaurant. We'd crossed paths by chance at an event a few weeks earlier and I was surprised by how much we had in common. She had a rare kind of quality about her that made me feel safe enough to be completely myself from the off.

Kate and I, however, hadn't spoken in months. A lot had happened to lead us there, and yet it still felt raw and unresolved.

As my friend poured a glass of wine, I found myself recounting the story of Kate, my hands gesturing as I tried to capture the essence of someone I had once been so close to, someone who had meant so much to me, yet whose presence still carried a lingering confusion.

'It's hard to put into words why you love someone, isn't it?' she said, pausing the small puppet show I seemed to have put on with my hands. I stopped mid-sentence and felt my eyes welling up as I placed my hands back down on the table beneath me.

I hadn't said anything about loving her, but somehow my feelings were transparent, and the sudden onset of vulnerability stung.

'I don't understand it,' I said, staring at my lap. 'I wish I had the words, but I don't.'

She looked back at me. 'Sometimes there isn't an answer. Sometimes, simply, your life wouldn't feel right without them. It's almost as if the answer lies in what it's not, rather than what it is, and it would be wrong *not* to love them.'

I looked back up at her.

'Well... f*ck,' I said. 'I guess we just found the words'.

For so long, I'd hoped Kate would reflect on her feelings and share them with me. For months, we had been stuck in a back-and-forth, sensing what lay beneath the surface but never fully voicing it.

But the confusion wasn't hers alone. Whenever I had tried to put into words what the connection truly meant, I skirted around the full truth, speaking in fragments, in ways that felt safer than admitting how I really felt.

And what followed was a barrage of questions I couldn't answer:

Why had I engaged in a dynamic that didn't belong to me?

Why had this stayed with me more deeply than any other relationship?

And what did I actually mean to her?

I had always encouraged others, no matter how scared they were, to put their cards on the table. Yet here I was, realising I had held everything back, becoming exactly what I used to urge others not to be. I wanted clarity. I wanted to tell the truth.

So what do you do if you find yourself in this situation?

You respect yourself enough to bring your feelings into the open – gently, honestly, without apology. You offer them not to control the outcome, but to free yourself from the weight of uncertainty.

And if she walks away, you let her.

But if she meets you there, maybe it wasn't a risk at all. Maybe it's the beginning.

Either way, naming your truth creates movement. It brings clarity, whether that leads to deepening the connection or finding the strength to step away. Neither path is easy, but staying stuck in the unknown, in that suspended grey space, is always harder.

You deserve peace. You deserve to know where you stand.

So I picked up the phone and I asked to meet.

How to gain clarity in the grey area

Clarity in the grey area between two women doesn't always arrive with tidy answers or definitive outcomes. More often, it's about learning to sit with uncertainty, recognising your emotions and understanding what they're really telling you. When a connection is undefined, clarity isn't always about labelling it, it's about tuning into yourself and choosing the path that feels most aligned, even if you don't have all the answers yet.

In this section, we'll explore why clarity can feel so elusive, and what internal patterns or external pressures might be clouding your perspective. You'll hear from other queer women who have navigated similar dynamics, reflect on what might need to be acknowledged, released or reimagined, and uncover what it truly means to move forwards with care, even when the way ahead isn't clear.

There isn't always a precise list of steps to follow in these situations, nor a script for how to move through a grey area with someone whose intentions or feelings are unclear. Often, the most powerful thing you *can* do is step back and understand the emotional dynamics at play, both theirs and yours. When you see the situation more clearly, you're better able to ask the important questions: *Is this connection serving me? Do I feel respected and seen? Do I want to keep investing, or is it time to let go?* Clarity doesn't always come from the other person. Sometimes it comes from choosing yourself, even when things are still a little blurry.

So let's take a look at five lessons that will help you understand yourself and the other person better – where you're coming from and what your behaviour means – so you can start to gain more clarity about what is going on.

Lesson 1: Nobody is perfect, but intention matters

Loving someone really is the scariest thing you can do. You put your heart in each other's hands and just hope the other person will take care of it. But sometimes, no matter how much trust exists between you, one or both of you drop it. Not necessarily out of cruelty, but out of fear, confusion or even emotional overwhelm.

When we feel let down by someone we deeply care for, it stings. We can swing between resentment, sadness, mistrust and anger. Sometimes those emotions take the lead, and we say or do things that don't reflect who we really are. And in the context of a grey-area connection between two women, where intimacy exists but definition doesn't, this volatility can be heightened. The space is already fragile, and one misstep can feel like everything is shattered.

I want to be clear: this is not about excusing or condoning harmful behaviour. The key is learning to distinguish between someone who is emotionally struggling but still acting with care, and someone who repeatedly crosses your boundaries or causes harm.

As queer women, we already carry the weight of societal marginalisation, so recognising mistreatment and knowing when to walk away is essential. Abuse, manipulation or violence should never be rationalised or tolerated. That said, we're all human, and we all make mistakes, especially in complex, emotionally charged situations.

In these grey-area dynamics, it's easy to confuse emotional overwhelm with intentional harm. But gaining clarity starts with learning to tell the difference. True care is reflected in someone's willingness to return to respect, honesty and accountability.

When you can recognise that, you stop waiting for mixed signals to make sense and start trusting your own intuition. And that's where clarity really begins.

To make peace in the grey area, try to separate hurt from harm. Ask yourself: *Is this person acting with intention to wound, or are they simply overwhelmed, confused or emotionally unprepared?* You don't have to excuse the impact, but recognising the difference can help release the grip of resentment.

If their actions still hurt, let yourself feel that but don't carry it as proof that you're unworthy or unlovable. Sometimes people can't meet you where you are, not because you asked for too much, but because they're not ready. That's not your fault and it doesn't always mean they meant to hurt you.

Lesson 2: Shift your perspective to understand others

You can't gain perspective while sitting inside your own head. Clarity doesn't come from zooming in: it comes from zooming out.

To truly understand what's going on between you and another woman, you need to look at the full picture: the circumstances, the environment, the emotions and the history. All of it matters. That kind of insight starts when you gently step outside of your own experience and try to imagine theirs.

Let me clarify this with an example:

If, as you're reading this, you're the one who feels grounded in your sexuality, and the connection you're navigating is with someone who isn't quite there yet, it's natural to feel powerless, because in many ways, you are.

Waiting for someone else to figure out how they feel or to finally put words to something that's unspoken can leave you feeling stuck on pause. It creates an invisible power dynamic, because while *you* might be ready to move forwards, they're still working out what direction they even want to go in. This imbalance can feel confusing and unfair.

But here's where a shift in perspective helps.

Not everyone is ready to hold space for their own feelings, let alone someone else's. And especially when it comes to sexuality, identity and desire, the process of 'figuring things out' can be messy, overwhelming and even painful. You might be eager for clarity but forcing someone into emotional growth before they're ready only builds resentment, and that's not a solid foundation for anything, especially not a relationship.

If they choose to engage, let it be from a place of choice, not pressure.

On the other hand, if you're the person reading this who *isn't* sure how you feel – perhaps you're the one in the proverbial driving seat and unsure how you got there – know this: you might not even realise the weight you're holding.

You may feel guilty, conflicted or torn between care and fear, and that's OK. Working through those feelings is valid, and necessary.

But again, shift the perspective.

While it's important to give yourself space to process, remember there's someone else on the other side of that silence, someone who likely cares an awful lot about you, who might be uncertain or confused about how you truly feel. You don't have to have all the answers, but if part of you knows that this person matters, that they're *not* just another connection but something rare and real, then let them know. Don't wait until they've walked away to realise you may have shared something most people spend a lifetime searching for.

Clarity doesn't always mean certainty. Sometimes it simply means being honest about where you are, what you feel and what you hope for, even if it's messy or imperfect.

Because the longer you sit in indecision, the more likely it is that the space between you grows into something neither of you knows how to bridge. Connection can only hold out for so long without being met halfway.

The clarity you're seeking won't arrive loudly: it won't shout. But it *will* speak, softly and steadily, if you give yourself the space to hear it.

When the noise settles and the distractions fade, the answers will come, and when they do, you'll know what's truly right for you.

Lesson 3: Understand what you're both carrying

When you begin to unpack a deep connection with another woman, especially one that sits in the uncertain space between friendship and romance, you're not just dealing with what's happening in the moment, you're also navigating a whole history of internalised messages, unspoken fears and past experiences that shape how both of you relate to closeness, desire and emotional safety.

For queer women, this can be particularly complex. Many of us have grown up questioning the legitimacy of our feelings, wondering if we're 'reading too much into it', if it's safe to say what we want or even if we're allowed to want more at all. Whether it's because of family, religion, culture or the subtle policing of emotions by heteronormative norms, these pressures don't just disappear when we meet someone we're drawn to. Instead, they sit quietly beneath the surface, until something awakens them.

And when that happens, it can activate our attachment systems – the emotional blueprint we each carry that shapes how we seek (or avoid) intimacy, reassurance and connection. Understanding your attachment style (*see* p. 178) and being curious about hers, too, can give you essential insight into *why* you're reacting the way you are, whether it's pulling away, clinging on, shutting down or overthinking every interaction. It can also help you separate *what's happening between you* from *what's being stirred up within you*. That distinction is often the key to finding clarity in the grey area, to recognise what's real, what's rooted in fear and what actually needs to be said.

Lesson 4: Understand that distance doesn't always equal rejection

When someone creates distance, it can feel like a direct rejection of you, your emotions or the connection you thought you shared. But stepping back isn't always about disinterest or avoidance. Sometimes it's simply the only way that person knows how to manage what they're feeling. They might be emotionally overwhelmed, unsure how to engage with the situation or reluctant to face the discomfort it brings. And while that can feel painful, it's still their choice. Not everyone has the tools or the emotional capacity to sit in discomfort and face things head-on. Recognising this doesn't make the hurt disappear, but it can offer a sense of peace, and a little more compassion for both you and them.

Most of us, wherever we land on the attachment spectrum, try to manage emotional overwhelm in the ways we've learned to survive.

Some people become fixated on resolution, seeking clarity, reassurance or explaining their feelings over and over again. Others retreat inwards, shut down and convince themselves it never mattered in the first place.

The cycle in the grey area can often look like this:

- **Emotions arise** – A moment shifts the dynamic between two people and suddenly things feel more charged than either person expected.
- **One person, or both, senses the emotional stakes** – This could be the realisation that feelings are developing or getting too deep. Either way, it feels vulnerable, and that vulnerability sets off alarm bells.
- **An instinctive pull-back happens** – One person distances themselves, maybe subtly, maybe abruptly. They stop texting back as quickly, cancel plans or retreat into silence.
- **Confusion takes hold** – The other person feels the shift but doesn't understand it. They question themselves: *Did I do something wrong? Did I imagine the whole thing?*
- **The connection gets minimised** – Someone downplays what happened: 'It wasn't that deep', 'We were just friends', 'I was confused'. This isn't necessarily dishonesty; it's often a way to manage discomfort.
- **Emotional overwhelm is avoided but not resolved** – On the surface, the tension might settle. But underneath, the feelings haven't gone away – they've just been buried.

This is the cycle many people, especially queer women in undefined or emotionally ambiguous connections, get caught in. Because when the feelings are real but the situation is unclear, it can feel easier to retreat than to risk what comes with being honest.

But avoidance doesn't erase emotional truth. It only delays the clarity we're really craving and covers up the fear that's hiding underneath. Fear of being vulnerable. Fear of losing something precious. Fear of opening a door that might be impossible to close once you walk through it.

Throughout this book, we've seen that people pull away for all kinds of reasons. Maybe they don't think they deserve to be loved that well, and the vulnerability overwhelms them. Maybe someone else is involved.

Maybe they care deeply but aren't ready to face it. Or maybe . . . they simply don't know where to start.

Whatever the reason, it hurts. But remember this:

Just because someone chooses not to stay, it doesn't mean the connection wasn't real.

People don't usually run unless there's something *real* to run from.

So why do people push away the ones they love?

More often than not, it comes down to fear – and not just any fear, but the fear of *abandonment*. The fear of being left behind, of not being chosen, of not being loved in the way we truly need.

Yes, this kind of fear is often linked to avoidant attachment styles, but let's be real: it's universal. It doesn't matter how self-aware or emotionally intelligent you are. Anyone can reject closeness when it feels like that closeness might eventually be taken away.

So what do we do? We protect ourselves, we pull back and we close the door, before someone else has the chance to close it on us first. We tell ourselves we're being smart, staying one step ahead of heartbreak. But often, what we're really doing is cutting off a connection that was never actually in danger. And in doing so, we don't just hurt ourselves, we hurt the person who may have had no intention of leaving at all.

But here's the irony of this grey area, especially in connections between two women. Both people are usually craving the same thing:

Reassurance.

Reassurance that the feelings are mutual, that they're not imagining it, and that saying it out loud won't scare the other person away.

But for any connection to survive, it takes more than silent wishing. It takes *two* people willing to be brave, *two* people willing to stay, even when it gets uncomfortable and *two* people who choose not to run, even when they're scared.

So if you're feeling stuck, whether you're the one holding on or pulling away, remember this:

Just because someone leaves doesn't mean it wasn't real.

And just because you're afraid doesn't mean you're not ready. You might never feel fully ready; most of us don't. But the clarity you're seeking only begins the moment you stop avoiding your truth.

Lesson 5: Don't chase their shadow

A few months after Kate and I stopped talking, I found myself standing outside a pub in Notting Hill in London with someone new. She held her drink delicately, bangs of hair falling across her face, in a way that felt nostalgic. She lit a cigarette and stared back at me.

'I want to kiss you,' she said.

'So kiss me,' I replied.

Twenty-four hours later, I regretted dropping that line.

I don't know if it was the universe trying to send me a lesson or just a strange coincidence that weekend, but it left me wondering: why do we chase people who feel like someone we've lost?

Turns out, there's psychological research behind that pull.

The *transference effect* suggests many of us unconsciously seek out partners who resemble our exes (or even our parents!). We're drawn to traits that feel familiar, comforting and safe. Similarly, the *similarity-attraction theory* suggests we're drawn to people who reflect our own values, personality traits and behaviours, even when that means repeating patterns we thought we'd left behind.

It's part biology, part comfort and part unresolved emotional history.

For queer women especially, where relationship scripts are often unclear or non-existent, the pull towards something familiar can feel even more intense. Without the traditional road map, we sometimes mistake resemblance for resonance, or chemistry for connection.

But here's the thing: just because a person *feels* familiar, like someone you once cared about, it doesn't mean the connection is the same. Real connection isn't built on surface familiarity – it's built on chemistry, emotional safety, depth and reciprocity.

And that was the real lesson.

Everyone tells you to move on quickly, to get over it, start fresh and find someone new, but it doesn't always work like that. Especially not for queer women navigating complex emotional terrain.

It's OK to wait and to not move on too quickly, to not settle for the first thing that comes along just because the last thing remains undefined or didn't work out, and to honour what was real instead of replacing it with something that simply *looks* right from the outside.

Because what you're really waiting for, and what you fully deserve, is a connection that makes you feel alive, safe and *seen*.

To explore how others have navigated these lessons, I asked my community of queer women to share their reflections on the ambiguous endings or new beginnings of grey area relationships: what they felt, what they learned and what helped them move forwards:

QUEER VOICES

'It was brutal because there are no clear rules. You lose a friend and a maybe-lover at once. The grief is real even when the relationship is undefined.'

'It hurts like a break-up, but in order to move on you have to acknowledge that there were unspoken feelings going on, and that can't continue.'

'For me it actually wasn't until we stopped talking that I realised how entangled we'd become. That pause gave us both the courage to come back and finally say what we'd been dancing around for months. So for me, it wasn't an end, more like a deep breath.'

'It was awful. I became rude, and angry. I was on holiday with her, we decided it wasn't working, so we agreed she would fly home a day earlier. But it was my actions that led to it, my insecurities – I couldn't communicate properly about how I felt and it led us there.'

'For me things came to a head, and we took a month apart. When we came back, we took a long walk and told each other what we wanted out of the relationship, and how that looked different than the status quo. It was the most cathartic conversation I've ever had.'

'Clarity is key. For me, it was completely cutting contact. It hurt like a b*tch but it was the best move. You need to grieve: the intensity was real, even if it never fit a neat box.'

MY STORY

Being around Kate again felt different. Nothing had changed, and yet everything had. We still laughed the way we used to, but there was a subtle distance, a tension I couldn't quite name. I didn't know what had happened in the months we hadn't spoken, what she had reflected on, and part of me still carries a quiet sadness for the gaps in the story I never got to understand.

In the end, I gave her a choice: to step towards me, even just a little, or to step away completely.

When it ended, it felt awful. I couldn't call it a break-up, because it was never officially a relationship to begin with, but it was sad, just the same.

You might assume I was angry afterwards, but I wasn't. Being part of the connection never hurt; it was losing it that did. And though it took me time to realise it, she hadn't rejected me – she had simply chosen not to step into the life that would have brought us together.

Kate knew me in ways other people didn't. She was proud of who I was, but more importantly, she believed in who I could become – a belief that still shapes me. I hope she'd recognise the parts of herself that still live on in me. Sometimes, though, the bravest thing we can do is keep becoming ourselves, even when the person who once knew us best isn't there to witness it.

Whatever it meant to each of us, I don't doubt there was care there. You don't share something like that with someone and not carry it with you – and I know I'd still pick up if she called.

The hardest part of concluding a connection in the grey area often isn't the ending itself, it's the almosts. The questions that linger when things don't end neatly, or when they are cut off in ways that aren't entirely mutual. It can leave you wondering how much of what was said – or left unsaid – was shaped by fear: fear of what the connection could have become if you had allowed it to grow.

But here's the truth. A connection never loses its meaning just because it was complicated, messy or ends without explanation. Sometimes, clarity doesn't come from a neat ending – it comes from seeing the truth of the choice, and finding your own peace within it.

Kate once told me she couldn't understand why I liked her. She thought I was blinded by the idea of who she could be, rather than who she truly was.

I didn't know how to answer her then, but if she asked me again, I'd say this:

We don't just fall in love with a person. We fall in love with how they make us *feel*.

They say to be loved is to be truly seen, and as much as I roll my eyes at clichés, that one annoyingly holds weight.

Because maybe it's only when you begin to feel the quiet ways someone holds you in their heart that you can begin to love who you are in *yours*. And what a rare kind of blessing it is, to understand the version of yourself that exists in someone else's story.

All I ever wanted was for Kate to see herself the way I saw her, but somewhere along the way, in trying to show her, I found myself instead.

Maybe that's the subtle miracle of being seen: not just that someone holds up a mirror to you, but that you finally recognise the reflection staring back.

Maybe *that's* the real lesson in all of this, that no matter how your story ends, time spent in the grey area can still leave you with something lasting: a deeper love for yourself, and for who you've become *because* of it.

I was never afraid of saying how I felt. I was only ever afraid that she'd never truly understand the depth to which I felt it. That even through all the grey areas, the ups and downs, and uncertainty, it helped me find a way back to myself.

And that kind of love, regardless of how long it lasts, leaves a mark that stays.

And for that, I'll always be grateful.

EIGHT

Closing thoughts

This book is a companion for the in between, that uncertain space between fear and freedom. Between hiding who you are and learning to live openly. Between surviving the expectations placed upon you and stepping into a life that feels truly your own.

It's about the messy, beautiful and sometimes painful process of owning your identity as a queer woman, and everything that comes with it.

As we've explored, healing and becoming don't happen just by *waiting*. They happen by *doing* – by asking the uncomfortable questions, having hard conversations and allowing yourself to be seen, even when you're not entirely sure how to explain who you are yet.

Action, no matter how small, is what transforms *reflection* into *momentum*.

It doesn't have to be big just yet. It might be:

- Coming out to one trusted friend
- Wearing what makes you feel like *you* for the first time
- Starting therapy
- Ending a relationship that's keeping you small
- Joining a community where you're not the only one in the room

These small steps are all powerful acts of resistance against a world that often wants us to stay invisible.

Of course, not everyone can just leap. You might be stuck in a situation you can't leave yet, living with family or a partner who for various reasons

CLOSING THOUGHTS

might not understand, in a relationship that doesn't reflect who you are, or you simply might not have the resources yet to make a change. If that's where you are currently at, know this: you don't have to rush. You don't have to burn it all down. But you can begin to imagine the life you want. You can start planning, dreaming and rebuilding from the inside out.

The life you want doesn't begin with placing one shaky brick on top of another, it starts by being brave and laying a solid foundation.

That foundation is *you*.

We often associate bravery with grand gestures or big moments of courage, but real bravery is quieter, and far more powerful. It's saying to yourself, *I'm not ready – but let's start anyway*. It's admitting, *This is terrifying – but let me be frightened for a while* and it's accepting, *I don't know how I'll get there – but the first step forwards is today*.

True bravery is radical honesty. It's dismantling the parts of you that no longer serve you and carefully rebuilding from a place of self-awareness and truth.

And what are we choosing bravery *for*?

Happiness.

Not the fleeting, performative kind, but the quiet, soul-deep kind.

For years, I misunderstood what happiness really meant. I thought it was about constant highs, external validation or ticking off milestones. But I've come to learn that true happiness is *peace*. It's being able to say 'I am who I am' and genuinely feel it, laughing with people who truly see you and waking up one morning and realising your life finally feels like it fits.

That kind of peace isn't a luxury or a far-off dream. It's something you *deserve*.

And it's sure as hell *worth* being brave for.

From the bottom of my heart, I truly hope that these pages have reminded you that you're not alone. That you're allowed to feel unsure and still move forwards and that your identity, your softness and your strength are all things to be proud of and celebrated, not feared.

I hope you feel empowered to own your truth, to speak it aloud, and to step fully into who you are.

Happiness is waiting for you, and you're allowed to claim it.

To round off this book, I asked a group of queer women who've walked this path before, through the uncertainty, the coming out, the transition and the rebuilding, to share what they wish someone had told them when they were in the in between.

Their words are here to remind you that you are never alone, even when it feels like it, and that community, connection and courage *are* within reach.

Take what resonates and bring it with you into the next stage of your life:

QUEER VOICES

'My therapist once asked me to imagine myself as a whole and complete cake, beautifully iced. A metaphor for being enough. Any future partner is simply the cherry on top: they add to the decadence, but they aren't the whole dessert. And if someone pinches the cherry off the top for a nibble, it doesn't diminish the wholeness of the cake beneath. That has stayed with me over the years – wholeness isn't something another person can give you: it's something you have to nurture and work on for yourself.'

'I'm not religious. I don't believe in fate. But what I do believe is that things tend to have a habit of eventually coming good. Sometimes times can be hard. But something good is coming. I promise.'

'Learn to find joy in change. You'll never run out of things to make you happy.'

'A lot of things aren't within our control, so learning to appreciate our experiences and trusting that everything works out eventually is really important.'

'Your journey doesn't need to mirror anyone else's. Trust your timing, honour your feelings and let yourself grow at your own pace. You are not too late, too much or too complicated – you are exactly enough.'

'Remember it's called a journey for a reason. Happiness is achievable but not without vulnerability and fear. You have to move through it.'

'You're not alone. There will be other women on similar journeys, those further ahead who can help you, those behind who you can help too.'

'You know yourself better than anyone else does. Make time to understand yourself and then trust your instincts.'

CLOSING THOUGHTS

'I have struggled with mental health and dark times for years, and I am still here – every dip is different and with every dip you do learn something different, that skin does get thicker, people really do come and go. Friends I have now are not the people I started the year with. I am a strong believer that things do happen for a reason, and what goes around comes around. Focus on things you can do: go to the gym, go for that walk, eat that snack. My favourite book is my passport: I use it wisely.'

'I used to write a list every day. I had to start with the basics: get out of bed, have a shower, eat. Once I ticked all three I added more until they weren't basic: hoover, go for a 5k walk, buy new jeans, join a group. I would congratulate myself for completing each task until it became normal to be part of the world. I still congratulate myself. Moving forwards is the only option.'

There is so much goodness to come, and the hard times are worth it

'Queerness is a journey, and it's going to take you on some wild rides, with some rides being harder than others! When things have been hard, I've thought of my past self, the self who felt like something was missing, that things didn't feel right, that wasn't her full self but couldn't put their finger on why. I know I would much rather be dealing with the hardships that come with being my truest, fullest version of myself than who I was stuck as before. For every low, there is a high: cool things you may not have done before you came out and a load of firsts you haven't experienced yet. There is so much goodness to come, and the hard times are worth it to experience that queer joy.'

'The past is history, the future is a mystery, so we live for today.'

A FINAL STORY FROM ME

In July 2025 I threw some clothes into a suitcase, boarded a flight to Iceland and set out to host a trip for 13 queer women I'd never met before.

I hadn't gone into the week with any intention beyond creating a space for others to connect, yet somewhere along the way, the final piece of my own puzzle quietly fell into place.

One afternoon, after lacing on ice shoes, 12 layers of waterproof clothing and hard hats, we began a slow ascent up a glacier, one by one, in a line, holding hands as we climbed.

Not only was it a test of strength, but more importantly, a test of community. Because when we reached the top, exhausted but exhilarated, we realised we'd done something we hadn't known we were capable of.

We had conquered a complete unknown.

And we had done it together.

Back in the bus, all of us completely soaked to our underwear, drenched in sweat, mud and rain, had smiles across our faces, and laughing louder than I'd ever laughed before, something hit me.

I looked around at this group of beautiful women I'd brought together, strangers just days earlier, and felt something I had never truly felt: the deepest sense of complete belonging.

Not just with them, but perhaps most importantly, with *myself*.

It had been nearly two decades since I had sat in a classroom aged 15, where my journey with my sexuality began, wondering if I'd ever feel happy enough to experience a life that I knew I so desperately wanted, but didn't think I deserved.

I never imagined back then what the future me would look like, because I couldn't comprehend that I would be happy enough to find her at all.

But suddenly in the middle of nowhere, on a bus full of strangers whose prescence felt like home, there she was. Thirty-one years old and beyond grateful that I'd flipped the script, changed the narrative and chosen a life that closed the door on what was, to make space for what could be.

And what a powerful gift to give yourself, to choose a life that lights you up.

People are right when they say these things hit you out of nowhere. A random Tuesday in mid-July, now forever a reminder of a journey full of ups and downs, struggle, hope and growth.

A moment that indeed will stay with me *forever*.

CLOSING THOUGHTS

It might take a few months, a few years or even a few decades but I believe that a moment like this is waiting out there for you too.

You can't predict the future, but you can take control of the present and have faith in the journey.

What is meant for you will *always* find you; you just need to be brave enough to allow yourself to listen.

It might be the end of this book, but it's only the *beginning* of yours.

Don't be afraid to turn a new chapter.

Because who knows, you might *really* like the story that unfolds…

Acknowledgements

For my mum: There are no words to describe the depth of love I feel for you and the support you have shown me over the years. You have given me the duality of a softness that helps others feel seen and the fierceness to turn any dream I have into a reality. There are so many people out there who I know this book will help, but these pages are only possible because you showed me *first* what it means to truly love and be loved.

For my dad: Who I know will read this book cover to cover and think, *Christ, you've only mentioned me twice, and one of those times was in reference to a Dido CD.* This book is only possible because you taught me how to master the art of humour and wordplay, and for that I owe you the biggest credit, because the world would be dull as hell if you hadn't shown me how to see it.

For my friends: You have all held my hand through thick and thin, no matter what version of myself shows up or however lost, confused and alone I've felt. Some days we dance through life with laughter and some days with pain, but we are always stronger for it. I hope everyone can experience the kind of love we share, and that this book will bring the possibility of such beautiful connections to others.

For my online audience: You are the reason why I am so fierce in my belief that change is possible. Thank you for believing in my dream to make the queer space uplifting, connected and joyful for all. Although I can't talk to you directly, just know that I am beyond grateful for each and every one of you and your support carries me and pushes me forward *every day*.

ACKNOWLEDGEMENTS

For the strangers I've crossed paths with: I will never forget the way you made me feel and the nuggets of wisdom I've received. Your kindness has fallen on me like glitter and helped me to shine brighter than I ever imagined. The moments we shared, the conversations we had and the way that we held each other's hands as we walked each other part of the way home, and back to ourselves, have made a lasting footprint in my soul and for that I will forever be grateful.

For the people I have loved: You know who you are as you turn these pages. You have helped shape parts of me that nobody else will ever know or touch. What we shared is etched deep in my memories, where it will live regardless of the time and space between us. Some of our love was fleeting, and some forever lasting. Either way I have been shaped, held and moved by it, and I exist to tell these stories because of what held me up along the way: you.

This isn't just my story, it's a tapestry woven from the lives of everyone who's touched mine, and those who I am yet to meet.

Every person I've crossed paths with has left a mark, shaping who I am today.

And the same goes for you.

Connection is one of the most *powerful* things we have. We're always stronger when we choose to let others in, lead with kindness and fully embrace the life we've been given.

Remember: life is not a dress rehearsal: it's the real deal. So please live it.

Sources

Chapter 1 – Coming Out

15 **'10% of LGBTQ+ adults in the U.S. come out after age 30':** McCarthy, J., 'LGBTQ+ Adults Are Coming Out at Younger Ages Than in the Past', *Gallup*, 26 July 2024. Available at: https://news.gallup.com/poll/647636/lgbtq-adults-coming-younger-ages-past.aspx

15 **'52% came out after the age of 18':** Rico, M., 'The generational shift in LGBTQI women "coming out"', *Kantar*, 22 April 2020. Available at: www.kantar.com/Inspiration/Equality/The-generational-shift-in-LGBTQI-women-coming-out

15 **many older adults not fully coming out until well into their 20s:** Grace, G., 'Why are more women opting to date women in their 40s?', *Body+Soul*, 6 March 2024. Available at: www.bodyandsoul.com.au/relationships/why-are-more-women-coming-out-as-lesbians-in-their-50s/image-gallery/0d13aecd36d3bb7ccfa0894bff39724a

23 **This is part of what psychologists call 'negativity bias':** Romm, A., 'Negativity Bias: Why We Expect the Worst and How to Change That', *Aviva Romm*, 12 October 2022. Available at: https://avivaromm.com/negativity-bias/

23 **Certain parts of our brain are highly sensitive to danger cues:** Mobbs, D., Hagan, C.C., Dalgleish, T., Silston, B. and Prévost, C., 'The ecology of human fear: survival optimization and the nervous system', *Frontiers in Neuroscience*, 18 March 2015. Available at: www.frontiersin.org/journals/neuroscience/articles/10.3389/fnins.2015.00055

and Flannelly, K.J., Koenig, H.G., Galek, K. and Ellison, C.G., 'Beliefs, mental health, and evolutionary threat assessment systems in the brain', *Journal of Nervous and Mental Disease*, December 2007. Available at: https://pubmed.ncbi.nlm.nih.gov/18091193/

27 **when stress becomes chronic, cortisol can do more harm than good:** Mayo Clinic Staff, 'Chronic stress puts your health at risk', *Mayo Clinic*, 1 August 2023. Available at: www.mayoclinic.org/healthy-lifestyle/stress-management/in-depth/stress/art-20046037

27 **Too much of it disrupts sleep:** Wright, K.P. Jr, Drake, A.L., Frey, D.J., Fleshner, M., DeSouza, C.A., Gronfier, C. and Czeisler, C.A., 'Influence of Sleep Deprivation and Circadian Misalignment on Cortisol, Inflammatory Markers, and Cytokine Balance', *Brain, Behavior, and Immunity*, July 2015. Available at: https://pmc.ncbi.nlm.nih.gov/articles/PMC5401766

and Thompson, K.I., Chau, M., Lorenzetti, M.S., Hill, L.D., Fins, A.I. and Tartar, J.L., 'Acute sleep deprivation disrupts emotion, cognition, inflammation, and cortisol in young healthy adults', *Frontiers in Behavioral Neuroscience*, 23 September 2022. Available at: https://pubmed.ncbi.nlm.nih.gov/36212194/

31 **Analysis paralysis is a state where conflicting thoughts and emotions crash:** Boogaard, K., 'How to get unstuck: tips for moving past analysis paralysis', *Atlassian*, 5 January 2024. Available at: www.atlassian.com/blog/productivity/analysis-paralysis

SOURCES

and Harrison, T., 'What Causes Analysis Paralysis? 7 Factors That Keep You From Making Decisions', *Mind Journal*, no date. Available at: https://themindsjournal.com/what-causes-analysis-paralysis-7-factors-that-keep-you-from-making-decisions

and Clarke, J., 'What Is Analysis Paralysis?', *Verywell Mind*, 27 November 2023. Available at: www.verywellmind.com/what-is-analysis-paralysis-5223790

Chapter 2 – Labels

50 **why the Kinsey Scale made such an impact:** 'Kinsey Scale Score Explained: Your Comprehensive Guide to Each Number (0–6)', Kinseyscale.org. Available at: https://kinseyscale.org/blog/kinsey-scale-score-explained-your-comprehensive-guide-to-each-number-0-6

51 **'one in three now use "nontraditional labels" . . .':** Porta, C.M., Gower, A.L., Brown, C., Wood, B. and Eisenberg, M.E., 'Perceptions of Sexual Orientation and Gender Identity Minority Adolescents About Labels', *Western Journal of Nursing Research*, 42(2), February 2020, 81–89. Available at: https://pubmed.ncbi.nlm.nih.gov/30943875/

Chapter 3 – Connections

72 **deliberately introduce positive experiences or reminders of joy:** Emmons, R.A. and McCullough, M.E., 'Counting blessings versus burdens: An experimental investigation of gratitude and subjective well-being in daily life', *Journal of Personality and Social Psychology*, 84(2), 2003, 377–389. Available at: https://psycnet.apa.org/doiLanding?doi=10.1037%2F0022-3514.84.2.377

74 **linked to our cognition, memory and emotional processing:** Moore, S.T., Hirasaki, E., Raphan, T. and Cohen, B., 'The human vestibulo-ocular reflex during linear locomotion', *Annals of the New York Academy of Sciences*, 942, October 2001, 139–147. Available at: https://pubmed.ncbi.nlm.nih.gov/11710456/

74 **influence memory vividness and emotionality:** Jarrett, C., 'Improve Your Memory: Wiggle Your Eyes Back and Forth', *British Psychological Society Research Digest*, 26 March 2007. Available at: www.bps.org.uk/research-digest/improve-your-memory-wiggle-your-eyes-back-and-forth

74 **A meta-analysis by Houben *et al.*:** Houben, S.T.L., Otgaar, H., Roelofs, J., Merckelbach, H., Muris, P., 'The effects of eye movements and alternative dual tasks on the vividness and emotionality of negative autobiographical memories: A meta-analysis of laboratory studies', *Journal of Experimental Psychopathology*, 11(1), 2020. Available at: https://journals.sagepub.com/doi/10.1177/2043808720907744

76 **Early humans relied on pooling resources, co-operative hunting and collective protection:** Nowak, M.A. and Highfield, R., *SuperCooperators: Altruism, Evolution, and Why We Need Each Other to Succeed* (Free Press, 2011).

77 **the 'tend and befriend' response:** Taylor, S.E., Klein, L.C., Lewis, B.P., Gruenewald, T.L., Gurung, R.A.R. and Updegraff, J.A., 'Biobehavioral responses to stress in females: Tend-and-befriend, not fight-or-flight', *Psychological Review*, 107(3), 2000, 411–429. Available at: https://psycnet.apa.org/doiLanding?doi=10.1037%2F0033-295X.107.3.411

Chapter 4 – Dating

89 **tend to report more emotional support:** Joyner, K., Manning, W. and Prince, B., 'The Qualities of Same-Sex and Different-Sex Couples in Young Adulthood', *Journal of Marriage and Family*, 81(2), April 2019, 487–505. Available at: https://pmc.ncbi.nlm.nih.gov/articles/PMC6516865/

89 **Part of this comes down to biology:** Becker, J.B., et al., *Sex Differences in the Brain: From Genes to Behavior* (Oxford University Press, 2019).

95 **the love languages framework outlined by Dr Gary Chapman:** Chapman, G., *The Five Love Languages: How to Express Heartfelt Commitment to Your Mate* (Northfield Publishing, 1992).

97 **In the 2023 OPEN survey:** OPEN (Organization for Polyamory and Ethical Non-monogamy), '2023 Community Survey Report', *OPEN*, 1 August 2023. Available at: www.open-love.org/blog/2023-community-survey-report

97 **Rubel and Burleigh's 2020 study:** Rubel, A.N. and Burleigh, T.J., 'Counting polyamorists who count: Prevalence and definitions of an under-researched form of consensual nonmonogamy', *Sexualities*, 23(1–2), 2018, 3–27. Available at: https://journals.sagepub.com/doi/10.1177/1363460718779781

99 **women generally want to see other women laughing:** Provine, R. R., *Laughter: A Scientific Investigation* (Penguin Books, 2000).

105 **David Brooks talks about the concept of really leaning into listening:** Brooks, D., *How to Know a Person: The Art of Seeing Others Deeply and Being Deeply Seen* (Random House, 2023).

105 **Studies show that when people spend close time together:** Nikos-Rose, K. 'Lovers' hearts beat in sync, UC Davis study says', *UC Davis*, 8 February 2013. Available at: https://www.ucdavis.edu/news/lovers-hearts-beat-sync-uc-davis-study-says

and Helm J.L., Sbarra D., Ferrer E. 'Assessing cross-partner associations in physiological responses via coupled oscillator models', *Emotion*, 12 August 2012. doi: 10.1037/a0025036. Available at: http://www.ncbi.nlm.nih.gov/pubmed/21910541

and Coutinho, J., Pereira, A., Oliveira-Silva, P., Meier, D., Lourenço, V., & Tschacher, W. (2021). 'When our hearts beat together: Cardiac synchrony as an entry point to understand dyadic co-regulation in couples.' *Psychophysiology*, 58(3), e13739. https://doi.org/10.1111/psyp.13739

105 **studies show that when people spend time close together:** Proverbio, A.M., Zani, A. and Adorni, R., 'Neural markers of a greater female responsiveness to social stimuli', *BMC Neuroscience*, 30 June 2008. Available at: https://bmcneurosci.biomedcentral.com/articles/10.1186/1471-2202-9-56   https://pmc.ncbi.nlm.nih.gov/articles/PMC2819096/https://pubmed.ncbi.nlm.nih.gov/25090107/

108: **Psychologists point out that asking questions (especially follow-ups) signals curiosity:** Leyba, E., 'Why Everyone Should Ask More Questions on Dates', *Psychology Today*, 9 February 2024. Available at: www.psychologytoday.com/gb/blog/joyful-parenting/202401/what-science-says-about-asking-questions-on-a-date

108 **When we're nervous we tend to talk shit:** Reality Pathing, 'Why Do People Talk More When They're Nervous?', *Reality Pathing*, 10 July 2025. Available at: https://realitypathing.com/why-do-people-talk-more-when-theyre-nervouswww.verywellmind.com/do-their-nervous-habits-mean-they-like-me

SOURCES

109 Nervousness triggers the body's stress response: Huntington, C., 'Nervousness: Definition, Symptoms, & Relief', The Berkeley Well-Being Institute. Available at: www.berkeleywellbeing.com/nervousness www.bustle.com/p/7-unexpected-signs-you-give-off-nervous-energy

and 'Leading psychologist educating public about involuntary nervous reactions', *Mancunian Matters*, 19 September 2023. Available at: www.mancunianmatters.co.uk/news/19092023-leading-psychologist-educating-public-about-involuntary-nervous-reactions **remembering romantic details is closely tied:** Aydin, C., & Buyukcan-Tetik, A., 'Remembering the romantic past: Autobiographical memory functions and romantic relationship quality.' *PloS one*, 16(5), 2021, e0251004. https://doi.org/10.1371/journal.pone.0251004

and Holmberg, D., Thibault, T. M., & Pringle, J. D., 'Gender differences in romantic relationship memories: who remembers? Who cares?.' *Memory (Hove, England)*, 26(6), 816–830. 2018. Available at: https://pubmed.ncbi.nlm.nih.gov/29239695/

and Guilbault, V., & Philippe, F. L., 'Commitment in romantic relationships as a function of partners' encoding of important couple-related memories.' *Memory (Hove, England)*, 25(5), 2017, 595–606. Available at: https://pubmed.ncbi.nlm.nih.gov/27310766/

109 reported more vivid and detailed memories: Holmberg, D., Thibault, T.M. and Pringle, J.D., 'Gender differences in romantic relationship memories: who remembers? Who cares?', *Memory*, 26(6), July 2018, 816–830. Available at: https://pubmed.ncbi.nlm.nih.gov/29239695/

110 women tend to be more attuned to detail: Hall, J.A. and Schmid Mast, M., 'Are Women Always More Interpersonally Sensitive Than Men? Impact of Goals and Content Domain', *Personality and Social Psychology Bulletin*, 34(1), 2008, 144–155. (Original work published 2008). Available at: https://journals.sagepub.com/doi/abs/10.1177/0146167207309192

110 interpreting and recalling emotionally relevant cues: Mast, M.S. and Hall, J.A., 'Women's advantage at remembering others' appearance: A systematic look at the why and when of a gender difference', *Personality and Social Psychology Bulletin*, 32(3), March 2006, 353–364. Available at: https://pubmed.ncbi.nlm.nih.gov/16455862/https://pubmed.ncbi.nlm.nih.gov/22039333/

110 women outperform men in facial and visual memory tasks: Guilbault, V., & Philippe, F. L., 'Commitment in romantic relationships as a function of partners' encoding of important couple-related memories.' *Memory (Hove, England)*, 25(5), 2017, 595–606. Available at: https://pubmed.ncbi.nlm.nih.gov/27310766/

and Andreano, J.M. and Cahill, L., 'Sex influences on the neurobiology of learning and memory', *Cold Spring Harbor Laboratory Press*, 2009. Available at: http://www.learnmem.org/cgi/doi/10.1101/lm.918309.

and Rehnman, J., & Herlitz, A., 'Women remember more faces than men do.' *Acta psychologica*, 124(3), 344–355. 2007. https://doi.org/10.1016/j.actpsy.2006.04.004

110 True smiles and genuine laughter: Kraut, R.E. and Johnston, R.A., 'Social and emotional messages of smiling: An ethological approach', *Journal of Personality and Social Psychology*, 37(9), 1979, 1539–1553. Available at: https://psycnet.apa.org/doiLanding?doi=10.1037%2F0022-3514.37.9.1539

110 Neuroscience even shows that laughter releases endorphins and oxytocin: Dunbar, R. I., Baron, R., Frangou, A., Pearce, E., van Leeuwen, E. J., Stow, J., Partridge, G., MacDonald, I., Barra, V., & van Vugt, M. (2012). 'Social laughter is correlated with an elevated pain threshold.' *Proceedings. Biological sciences*, 279(1731), 1161–1167. https://doi.org/10.1098/rspb.2011.1373

and Manninen, S., Tuominen, L., Dunbar, R. I., Karjalainen, T., Hirvonen, J., Arponen, E., Hari, R., Jääskeläinen, I. P., Sams, M., & Nummenmaa, L., 'Social Laughter Triggers Endogenous Opioid Release in Humans', *The Journal of neuroscience: the official journal of the Society for Neuroscience*, 37(25), 2017, 6125–6131. https://doi.org/10.1523/JNEUROSCI.0688-16.2017

111 **this behaviour is a form of *preening*:** 'Preening', Changing Minds, Available at: changingminds.org/techniques/body/core_patterns/preening

112 **eyebrow flashes can foster connection:** Wilson, Edward O. "The Evolution of Communication." *Science*, vol. 176, no. 4035, 1972, pp. 625–27. *JSTOR*, http://www.jstor.org/stable/1734473. Accessed 3 Dec. 2025.

and Barash, David P., 'Human Ethology and Human Sociobiology.' *Behavioral and Brain Sciences* 2.1 (1979): 26–27. doi.org/10.1017/S0140525X00060428

112 **Some studies indicate that we emit and respond to subtle chemical cues:** Idan Frumin, I. et al., 'A social chemosignaling function for human handshaking', *eLife* **4**:e05154, 2015. https://doi.org/10.7554/eLife.05154

and Mutic S, Moellers EM, Wiesmann M and Freiherr J (2016) 'Chemosensory Communication of Gender Information: Masculinity Bias in Body Odor Perception and Femininity Bias Introduced by Chemosignals During Social Perception.', *Front. Psychol.* 6:1980. doi: 10.3389/fpsyg.2015.01980

and Wisman, A., & Shrira, I. (2020). Sexual Chemosignals: Evidence that Men Process Olfactory Signals of Women's Sexual Arousal. *Archives of sexual behavior*, 49(5), 1505–1516. https://doi.org/10.1007/s10508-019-01588-8

and Lübke, K. T., & Pause, B. M. (2015). Always follow your nose: the functional significance of social chemosignals in human reproduction and survival. *Hormones and behavior*, 68, 134–144. https://doi.org/10.1016/j.yhbeh.2014.10.001

and de Groot, J. H., Smeets, M. A., Kaldewaij, A., Duijndam, M. J., & Semin, G. R. (2012). Chemosignals communicate human emotions. *Psychological science*, 23(11), 1417–1424. https://doi.org/10.1177/0956797612445317

112 **deep breath helps regulate these physical responses:** Brown, R.P. and Gerbarg, P.L., '*Sudarshan Kriya* yogic breathing in the treatment of stress, anxiety, and depression: Part II—clinical applications and guidelines', *Journal of Alternative and Complementary Medicine*, 11(4), 2005, 711–717. Available at: https://www.researchgate.net/publication/7630254_Sudarshan_Kriya_Yogic_Breathing_in_the_Treatment_of_Stress_Anxiety_and_Depression_Part_II-Clinical_Applications_and_Guidelines

112 **Eye contact is one of the most powerful nonverbal cues:** Kellerman, J., Lewis, J. and Laird, J. D., 'Looking and loving: The effects of mutual gaze on feelings of romantic love'. *Journal of Research in Personality*, 23(2), 1989, 145–161. Available at: https://ia600607.us.archive.org/17/items/im-so.sexy/LookingAndLoving.pdf

113 **eye contact activates the brain's social and reward centres:** Conty, L., George, N. and Hietanen, J.K., 'Watching Eyes effects: When others meet the self', *Consciousness and Cognition*, 45, 2016, 184–197. Available at: www.researchgate.net/publication/308149096_Watching_Eyes_effects_When_others_meet_the_self

113 **deepen feelings of connection and attraction:** Hess, U., Blairy, S. and Kleck, R.E., 'The Influence of Facial Emotion Displays, Gender, and Ethnicity on Judgments of Dominance and Affiliation', *Journal of Nonverbal Behavior*, 24(4), 2000, 265–283. Available at: https://link.springer.com/article/10.1023/A:1006623213355

113 **their eyes move from one eye to the other:** Guéguen, N., 'Gaze and attraction: The "triangular gaze" pattern during flirting', *Journal of Social Psychology*, 155(1), 2015, 81–83.

SOURCES

113 **touch is one of the most powerful ways humans communicate:** Field, T., 'Touch for socioemotional and physical well-being: A review', *Developmental Review*, 2010. Available at: www.sciencedirect.com/science/article/abs/pii/S0273229711000025

and Gallace, A. and Spence, C., 'The science of interpersonal touch: An overview', *Neuroscience & Biobehavioral Reviews*, 34(2), 2010, 246–259. Available at: www.sciencedirect.com/science/article/abs/pii/S0149763408001723

124 **Anxiety and sexual tension are often two sides of the same coin:** Diamond, L.M., *The Oxford Handbook of Sexual and Gender Minority Mental Health* (Oxford University Press, 2017).

124 **people experiencing physiological arousal from fear or exercise:** Dutton, D.G. and Aron, A.P., 'Some evidence for heightened sexual attraction under conditions of high anxiety', *Journal of Personality and Social Psychology*, 30(4), 1974, 510–517. Available at: https://psycnet.apa.org/doiLanding?doi=10.1037%2Fh0037031

125 **studies on people who have been 'fake kidnapped':** Levenson, R.W., 'The autonomic nervous system and emotion'. In J. Cacioppo, L. Tassinary, and G. Berntson (Eds.), *Handbook of Psychophysiology* (Cambridge University Press, 2014).

Chapter 5 – Sex

135 **The words we use to describe sex have an interesting history:** Deczynski, R., 'Who Invented the Word "Sex" Anyway?', The Maudern, no date. Available at: www.getmaude.com/blogs/themaudern/etymology-of-sex

137 **Parents can also choose to withdraw their child from the teaching:** Department for Education, 'New RSHE Guidance: What It Means for Sex Education Lessons in Schools', Education Hub, 13 May 2024. Available at: www.educationhub.blog.gov.uk/2024/05/new-rshe-guidance-what-it-means-for-sex-education-lessons-in-schools

143 **According to a 2023 study by bedbible.com:** Bedbible, 'State of the Sex Toy Industry: Statistics and Trends', Bedbible, no date. Available at: www.bedbible.com/state-of-sex-toys-industry-statistics

144 **Reading Pornhub's '2024 Year In Review' report:** Pornhub Insights, '2024 Year In Review', Pornhub, 2024. Available at: www.pornhub.com/insights/2024-year-in-review#top-searches-pornstars

144 **there have been lengthy conversations around the ethics of it:** Prause, N. and Pfaus, J.G., 'Viewing Sexual Stimuli Associated with Greater Sexual Responsiveness, Not Erectile Dysfunction', *Frontiers in Psychology*, 6(1216), 2015. Available at: https://pubmed.ncbi.nlm.nih.gov/26185674/

145 **in the UK, almost 47 per cent of adults say health issues:** Royal College of Occupational Therapists, 'Almost half of UK adults' sex lives impacted by health problems', RCOT, 9 February 2024. Available at: www.rcot.co.uk/latest-news/sex-lives-impacted-health-problems

145 **up to one-third of adult women experience hypoactive sexual desire disorder:** Travers, C., 'Treatment of Hypoactive Sexual Desire Disorder', Verywell Health, 27 March 2024. Available at: www.verywellhealth.com/hypoactive-sexual-desire-disorder-symptoms-causes-diagnosis-treatment-and-coping-4767525

154 **Having sex on your period:** Frederick, D.A., 'Sexual Behaviour and Health Across the Menstrual Cycle', *Archives of Sexual Behavior*, 49(8), 2020, 2235–2247.

155 **studies have shown that orgasm releases endorphins and oxytocin:** Komisaruk, B.R., Beyer-Flores, C. and Whipple, B., *The Science of Orgasm* (Johns Hopkins University Press, 2006).

155 **libido can actually spike during menstruation:** Clayton, A.H. and Clift, J., 'Hormonal Influences on Female Sexual Desire', Obstetrics and Gynecology Clinics of North America, 48(4), 2021, 711–726.

155 **'around 30% of people report feeling more sexually aroused during their period':** Clue x Kinsey Institute, 'Sexual Behaviour and the Menstrual Cycle', Clue, 2018.

155 **it's important to practise safe sex:** 'Is It Safe to Have Sex During Your Period?', *Planned Parenthood*, 2022.

156 **'53% of lesbian and queer women have engaged in BDSM-related activities':** Kecojevic, A., Meleo-Erwin, Z.C., Basch, C. H. and Hammouda, M., 'A Thematic Analysis of Pre-Exposure Prophylaxis (PrEP) YouTube Videos', *Journal of Homosexuality*, 68(11), 2020, 1877–1898. Available at: www.tandfonline.com/doi/full/10.1080/00918369.2020.1712142

160 **nearly half of all women experience postcoital sadness at least once in their lives:** Schweitzer, R.D., O'Brien, J. and Burri, A., 'Postcoital Dysphoria: Prevalence and Psychological Correlates', *Sexual Medicine*, 3(4), December 2015, 244–253. Available at: https://pubmed.ncbi.nlm.nih.gov/26797056/

160 **postcoital crying can have many causes:** Vice, 'Crying After Sex: Why Emotions Surge Post-Orgasm', *Vice*, no date. Available at: www.vice.com/en/article/crying-emotions-after-sex-orgasm-in-relationships

161 **'Doing it once, I'm a philosopher; doing it twice, I'm a sodomite.':** Lehmiller, J., 'Is It Ever Just Sex', p. 131.

162 **about 90 per cent of cis women (and 50 per cent of cis men):** Nagoski, E., *Come As You Are: The Surprising New Science That Will Transform Your Sex Life* (Simon & Schuster, 2015).

162: **still having thoughts about men is totally normal regardless of your sexual orientation:** Anthony, C., 'Preferences for masculinity in male bodies change across the menstrual cycle', *Hormones and Behavior*, 2007. Available at: www.sciencedirect.com/science/article/abs/pii/S0018506X07000360?via%3Dihub

Chapter 6 – Relationships

169 **can also accelerate relationship milestones:** Diamond, L.M., Sexual Fluidity: Understanding Women's Love and Desire (Harvard University Press, 2008).

170 **common in LGBTQ+ populations due to experiences of marginalisation:** Katz-Wise, S.L. and Hyde, J.S., 'Victimization experiences of lesbian, gay, and bisexual individuals: A meta-analysis', Journal of Sex Research, 49(2–3), 2012, 142–167. Available at: https://psycnet.apa.org/record/2012-06003-004

170 **the importance of chosen family:** Weston, K., Families We Choose: Lesbians, Gays, Kinship (Columbia University Press, 1991).

174 **described continuing emotional ties and practical relationships with ex-partners:** Lahti, A., and Kolehmainen, M., 'LGBTIQ+ break-up assemblages: At the end of the rainbow', *Journal of Sociology*, 56(4), 2020, 608-628. Available at: https://doi.org/10.1177/1440783320964545

174 **'stay friends with their exes . . .':** Mogilski, J.K. and Welling, L.L.M., 'Staying friends with an ex: Sex and dark personality traits predict motivations for post-relationship friendship', *Personality and Individual Differences*, Volume 115, October 2017, 40–45. Available at: www.researchgate.net/profile/Justin-Mogilski/publication/303314151_Mogilski_2016

174 **a strong sign of emotional maturity:** Young, E., 'The Reasons We Stay Friends With an Ex', *Research Digest*, 8 June 2017. Available at: www.bps.org.uk/research-digest/reasons-we-stay-friends-ex

175 **couples who share core values:** van der Wal, R.C., Litzellachner, L.F., Karremans, J.C., Buiter, N., Breukel, J. and Maio, G.R., 'Values in Romantic Relationships', *Personality and Social Psychology Bulletin*, 50(7), July 2024, 1066–1079. Available at: https://pubmed.ncbi.nlm.nih.gov/36942922/

SOURCES

and Garcia, N., 'Why Values Shape Love and Happiness', *Enotalone*, 14 August 2023. Available at: www.enotalone.com/article/relationships/why-values-shape-love-and-happiness-r28413

175 a few of your fundamental values align: Gupta, S., '10 Signs You and Your Partner Are Compatible', Verywell Mind, 26 September 2025. Available at: www.verywellmind.com/signs-you-and-your-partner-compatible-7562809

and BetterHelp, 'What to Value in a Relationship? Common Core Values & the Importance of Shared Values', BetterHelp, updated 26 August 2025. Available at: www.betterhelp.com/advice/relations/what-to-value-in-a-relationship-common-core-values-the-importance-of-shared-values/

and Warner, R.C., 'Living in Alignment With Values, Identity, and Purpose', *Psychology Today*, 2 June 2025. Available at: www.psychologytoday.com/gb/blog/leadership-diversity-and-wellness/202506/living-in-alignment-with-values-identity-and-purpose

175 people in the queer community struggle with mental health complaints: The Trevor Project, 'Mental Health Diagnoses and Access to Care Among LGBTQ Young People', Research Briefs, 14 May 2025. Available at: www.thetrevorproject.org/research-briefs/mental-health-diagnoses-and-access-to-care-among-lgbtq-young-people/

175 Psychological research shows that couples who share core values: LaVarco, A. *et al.*, 'Self-Conscious Emotions and the Right Fronto-Temporal and Right Temporal Parietal Junction', Brain Sciences, 12(2), 2022, Article 138.

176 '65% report having at least one diagnosed mental health condition': Dey, M., 'LGBT Statistics by Employment, Education and Facts (2025)', *Sci-Tech Today*, 26 June 2025. Available at: www.sci-tech-today.com/stats/lgbt-statistics-updated

176 65% report having at least one diagnosed mental health condition: The Trevor Project, '2022 National Survey on LGBTQ Youth Mental Health', The Trevor Project, 2022. Available at: www.thetrevorproject.org/survey-2022

178 our attachment style can strongly impact: Mikulincer, M. and Shaver, P.R., *Attachment in Adulthood: Structure, Dynamics, and Change* (Guilford Press, 2007).

178 recent studies have begun to explore: Keskin, G., & Yig Itog Lu, G. T. (2021). 'The Effect of Early Traumatic Experiences on Attachment Styles in Sexual Gender Minority Individuals.' *Journal of forensic nursing*, 17(4), 219–228. https://doi.org/10.1097/JFN.0000000000000345

and Kardasz, Z., Gerymski, R., & Parker, A. (2023). 'Anxiety, Attachment Styles and Life Satisfaction in the Polish LGBTQ+ Community.' *International journal of environmental research and public health*, 20(14), 6392. https://doi.org/10.3390/ijerph2014639

and Trombetta, T., Fusco, C., Rollè, L., & Santona, A. (2025). Untangling Relational Ties: How Internalized Homonegativity and Adult Attachment Shape Relationship Quality in Lesbian and Gay Couples. *Behavioral sciences (Basel, Switzerland)*, 15(2), 205. https://doi.org/10.3390/bs15020205

and Cook, S. H., & Calebs, B. J. (2016). 'The Integrated Attachment and Sexual Minority Stress Model: Understanding the Role of Adult Attachment in the Health and Well-Being of Sexual Minority Men.' *Behavioral medicine (Washington, D.C.)*, 42(3), 164–173. https://doi.org/10.1080/08964289.2016.1165173

188 **Shame is more than just uncomfortable feelings:** Roth, L., Kaffenberger, T., Herwig, U. and Brühl, A.B., 'Brain activation associated with pride and shame', *Neuropsychobiology*, 69(2), 2014, 95–106. Available at: https://pubmed.ncbi.nlm.nih.gov/24577108/

188 **Psychological research shows that shame can lead to withdrawal:** Sznycer, D., Tooby, J., Cosmides, L., Porat, R., Shalvi, S. and Halperin, E., 'Shame closely tracks the threat of devaluation by others, even across cultures', Proceedings of the National Academy of Sciences of the United States of America, 113(10), 2016, 2625–2630. Available at: www.pnas.org/doi/full/10.1073/pnas.1514699113

188 **even physical symptoms:** Harris, C.R., 'Cardiovascular responses of embarrassment and effects of emotional suppression in a social setting', *Journal of Personality and Social Psychology*, 81(5), November 2001, 886–97. Available at: https://pubmed.ncbi.nlm.nih.gov/11708564/

and McGarity-Shipley, E., 'What a shame: Shame's Impact on arteries and health', The Physiological Society, 6 October 2022. Available at: www.physoc.org/blog/what-a-shame-shames-impact-on-arteries-and-health

and McGarity-Shipley, E.C., Lew, L.A., Bonafiglia, J.T. and Pyke, K.E., 'The acute effect of a laboratory shame induction protocol on endothelial function in young, healthy adults', *Experimental Physiology*, 107, 2022, 978–993. Available at: https://physoc.onlinelibrary.wiley.com/action/showCitFormats?doi=10.1113%2FEP090396

Chapter 7 – The grey area of love

208 **Women's sexuality is fluid:** Diamond, L.M., *Sexual Fluidity: Understanding Women's Love and Desire* (Harvard University Press, 2008).

and Ott, M.A., Corliss, H.L., Wypij, D., Rosario, M. and Austin, S.B., 'Sexual identity fluidity in young adults: Associations with sexual behavior and psychosocial variables', *Archives of Sexual Behavior*, 42(8), 2013, 1439–1446.

and Savin-Williams, R.C. and Vrangalova, Z., 'Mostly heterosexual as a distinct sexual orientation group: A review of the empirical evidence', *Developmental Review*, 33(1), 2013, 58–88. Available at: https://www.sciencedirect.com/science/article/abs/pii/S0273229713000026

208 **11.5% of women:** Geary, R. S., Tanton, C., Erens, B., Clifton, S., Prah, P., Wellings, K., Mitchell, K. R., Datta, J., Gravningen, K., Fuller, E., Johnson, A. M., Sonnenberg, P., & Mercer, C. H. (2018). Sexual identity, attraction and behaviour in Britain: The implications of using different dimensions of sexual orientation to estimate the size of sexual minority populations and inform public health interventions. *PloS one*, 13(1), e0189607. https://doi.org/10.1371/journal.pone.0189607

208 **'45% of younger women aged 17–34 reported…':** O'Connell, J., 'The Sex Survey: Same-sex attraction highest among women', *The Irish Times*, 29 June 2015. Available at: www.irishtimes.com/life-and-style/health-family/sex-survey/the-sex-survey-same-sex-attraction-highest-among-women-1.2266920

208 **a 1985 study revealed that 47%:** Coleman, E., 'Bisexual women in marriages', *Journal of Homosexuality*, 11(1–2), 1985, 87–99. Available at: https://pubmed.ncbi.nlm.nih.gov/4056398

210 **'roughly 30% of women reported shifts in their sexual identity over time':** Diamond, L.M., *Sexual Fluidity: Understanding Women's Love and Desire* (Harvard University Press, 2008).

211 **research shows that women are biologically inclined to respond by nurturing and connecting:** Gangestad, S., 'Female intrasexual competition and reputational effects on attractiveness among the Tsimane of Bolivia', *Evolution and Human Behavior*, 2005. Available at: www.sciencedirect.com/science/article/abs/pii/

SOURCES

S1090513805000577 www.ejog.org/article/S0301-2115(04)00352-5/abstract https://anatomypubs.onlinelibrary.wiley.com/doi/10.1002/ar.a.20133

212 **2. We're literally wired to 'tend and befriend':** Dess, N.K., 'Tend and Befriend', *Psychology Today*, September 2000. Available at: www.psychologytoday.com/gb/articles/200009/tend-and-befriend

and Sloan, E., 'Step Aside, Fight-or-Flight. "Tend and Befriend" Is Here to Help', SELF, 28 February 2025. Available at: www.self.com/story/tend-and-befriend-response

and University of California Los Angeles, 'UCLA Researchers Identify Key Biobehavioral Pattern Used By Women To Manage Stress', *ScienceDaily*, 22 May 2000. Available at: www.sciencedaily.com/releases/2000/05/000522082151.htm

and Taylor, S.E., Klein, L.C., Lewis, B.P., Gruenewald, T.L., Gurung, R.A.R. and Updegraff, J.A., 'Biobehavioral responses to stress in females: Tend-and-befriend, not fight-or-flight', *Psychological Review*, 107(3), 2000, 411–429. Available at: https://pubmed.ncbi.nlm.nih.gov/10941275

213 **68 per cent of romantic relationships begin as friendships:** Garcia, T., 'Two-thirds of couples start out as friends, research finds', *Guardian*, 12 July 2021. Available at: www.theguardian.com/lifeandstyle/2021/jul/12/two-thirds-of-couples-start-out-as-friends-research-finds

213 **if you identify as LGBTQ+, that number jumps to a whopping 85 per cent:** Factora, J., '85% of LGBTQ+ Relationships Started Out as Friends, According to Study', *Them*, 13 July 2021. Available at: www.them.us/story/85-percent-lgbtq-relationships-started-as-friendship-study

213 **Those friendships tend to simmer for almost two years before turning romantic:** Society for Personality and Social Psychology, 'Two-thirds of romantic couples start out as friends, study finds', 12 July 2021. Available at: https://phys.org/news/2021-07-two-thirds-romantic-couples-friends.html

218 **Oxford English Dictionary defines intimacy:** Oxford English Dictionary, 'Intimacy', *Oxford English Dictionary Online*, Oxford University Press, 2025. Available at: https://www.oed.com/dictionary/intimacy_n?tab=factsheet#132151

218 **The Interpersonal Process Model of Intimacy expands on this:** Laurenceau JP, Barrett LF, Pietromonaco PR. Intimacy as an interpersonal process: the importance of self-disclosure, partner disclosure, and perceived partner responsiveness in interpersonal exchanges. *J Pers Soc Psychol*. 1998 May; 74(5): 1238–51. doi: 10.1037//0022-3514.74.5.1238. PMID: 9599440.

220 **many studies have challenged the validity of this phenomenon:** Schmid, M.S., 'Are Women's Periods Synchronized for a Scientific Reason?', *SchmidScience*, 27 March 2025. Available at: https://schmidscience.com/are-women-s-periods-synchronized-for-a-scientific.html

220 **mirroring might look like sharing mannerisms:** Co-rumination. Wikipedia. Available at: https://en.wikipedia.org/wiki/Co-rumination

221 **Studies on non-verbal communication show:** Grammer, K., Kruck, K.B., Juette, A. and Fink, B., 'Nonverbal behavior in courtship: A survey', *Journal of Social and Personal Relationships*, 17 (4–5), 2000, 383–402. Available at: www.sciencedirect.com/science/article/abs/pii/S1090513800000532

221 **Any self-aware person knows what they're doing when they flirt:** Luscombe, B., 'The Science of Romance: Why We Flirt', *TIME Magazine*, 12 February 2008. Available at: https://time.com/archive/6683490/the-science-of-romance-why-we-flirt

221 **Studies on nonverbal communication:** Affiliative conflict theory. Wikipedia. Available at: https://en.wikipedia.org/wiki/Affiliative_conflict_theory

222 **Research on body language and behaviour:** Givens, D.B., 'Flirting Fascination', *Psychology Today*, 1 January 1999. Available at: www.psychologytoday.com/gb/articles/199901/flirting-fascination

and 'Romantic Body Language', *Changing Minds*. Available at: www.changingminds.org/techniques/body/romantic_body.htm

222 **It becomes more than friendship:** Marsh, W., 'Instant Signals She Likes You', Enotalone, no date. Available at: www.enotalone.com/article/relationships/attraction/instant-signals-she-likes-you-r28102

222 **Research on body language and behaviour:** Sexual Diversity, 'Body Language and Behavior Reveals Romantic Attraction', Sexual Diversity, no date. Available at: www.sexualdiversity.org/sexuality/love/409.php

223 **our brains release dopamine and oxytocin:** Acevedo, B.P., Aron, A., Fisher, H.E. and Brown, L.L., 'Neuroimaging of love: fMRI meta-analysis evidence toward new perspectives in sex, romance, and attachment', *Journal of Sex & Marital Therapy*, 37(4), 2011, 288–307. https://doi.org/10.1080/0092623X.2011.565177

223 **the brain's way of trying to define and solidify a connection:** McCraty, R., Atknson, M., Tomasino, D. and Bradley, R.T., 'The coherent heart: Heart-brain interactions, psychophysiological coherence, and the emergence of system-wide order', *Integral Review*, 5(2), 2009, 10–115. Available at: https://integral-review.org/issues/vol_5_no_2_mccraty_et_al_the_coherent_heart.pdf

225 **Psychologically, this limbo can keep our attachment systems activated long after:** Boss, P., *Ambiguous Loss: Learning to Live with Unresolved Grief* (Harvard University Press, 1999).

234 **unconsciously seek out partners who resemble our exes:** Taitz, S., 'Why Do We Choose Partners Who Remind Us of Past Wounds?', *Psychology Today*, 25 July 2023. Available at: www.psychologytoday.com/gb/blog/couples-thrive/202307/why-do-we-choose-partners-who-remind-us-past-wounds

and Schondelmayer, L., 'Do we actually prefer different characteristics in new romantic partners?', Department of Psychology, MSU, 2 August 2021. Available at: www.psychology.msu.edu/news-events/news/archives/2021/chopik-transference.html

the *similarity-attraction theory* **suggests:** Pennsylvania State University, 'The Similarity-Attraction Theory Means Harmony', Applied Social Psychology (PSU Blog), 13 April 2023. Available at: www.sites.psu.edu/aspsy/2023/04/13/the-similarity-attraction-theory-means-harmony